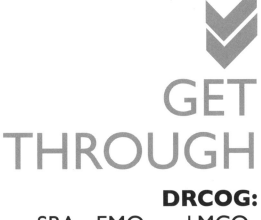

GET
THROUGH

DRCOG:
SBAs, EMQs and MCQs

D0492510

WITHDRAWN
FROM LIBRARY

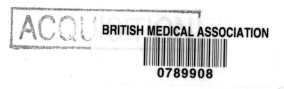

GET THROUGH

DRCOG:
SBAs, EMQs and MCQs

Rekha Wuntakal MB BS, MD, DNB, MRCOG, DFFP
Subspecialty Gynaecological Fellow, Department of Gynaecological
Oncology, Maidstone and Tunbridge Wells NHS Trust, Kent

Madhavi Kalidindi MRCOG
Consultant Obstetrician & Gynaecologist, Queen's Hospital,
BHR University Hospitals NHS Trust, London

Tony Hollingworth MB ChB, PhD, MBA, FRCS(Ed), FRCOG
Consultant in Obstetrics & Gynaecology, Whipps Cross Hospital,
Barts Health NHS Trust, London

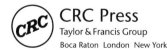

CRC Press
Taylor & Francis Group
Boca Raton London New York

CRC Press is an imprint of the
Taylor & Francis Group, an **informa** business

CRC Press
Taylor & Francis Group
6000 Broken Sound Parkway NW, Suite 300
Boca Raton, FL 33487-2742

© 2015 by Taylor & Francis Group, LLC
CRC Press is an imprint of Taylor & Francis Group, an Informa business

No claim to original U.S. Government works

Printed on acid-free paper
Version Date: 20140805

International Standard Book Number-13: 978-1-4822-1124-5 (Paperback)

Library of Congress Cataloging-in-Publication Data

Wuntakal, Rekha, author.
  Get through DRCOG : SBAs, EMQs and McQs / Rekha Wuntakal, Antony Hollingworth, Madhavi Kalidindi.
    p. ; cm. -- (Get through)
  Includes bibliographical references and index.
  ISBN 978-1-4822-1124-5 (hardcover : alk. paper)
    I. Hollingworth, Tony, author. II. Kalidindi, Madhavi, author. III. Title. IV. Series: Get through.
    [DNLM: 1. Gynecology--Examination Questions. 2. Obstetrics--Examination Questions. WP 18.2]

RG111
618.10076--dc23   2014027809

Visit the Taylor & Francis Web site at
http://www.taylorandfrancis.com

and the CRC Press Web site at
http://www.crcpress.com

CONTENTS

INTRODUCTION

The DRCOG examination is a test of knowledge of women's health care. The seven modules of the syllabus are basic clinical skills and basic surgical skills, antenatal care, management of labour and delivery, postpartum problems, gynaecological problems, plus fertility control. A thorough description of the topics covered in each of these modules is available on the Royal College of Obstetricians and Gynaecologists (RCOG) website: http://www.rcog.org.uk/education-and-exams/examinations/drcog/drcog-syllabus.

Format of the paper

The written paper is a 3-hour exam, and currently there is no OSCE exam. The time is equally divided between paper one and paper two.

Paper one consists of 30 extended matching questions (EMQs) and 18 single best answers (SBAs). Paper two is 200 five-part multiple choice questions (MCQs). There are a total of 350 marks, divided as follows:

EMQs – 105 marks (30%): Mark for each correct answer: 3.5
MCQs – 200 marks (57.1%): Mark for each correct answer: 1
SBAs – 45 marks (12.9%): Mark for each correct answer: 2.5

The RCOG website provides details about the format (http://www.rcog.org.uk/education-and-exams/examinations/drcog/drcog-format) with set examples for EMQs, SBAs and MCQs.

Extended matching questions (EMQs)

This section comprises 30 EMQs and each EMQ paper consists of 10 options with three questions: you need to match each question, statement or clinical scenario with one of the 10 options available. The questions are of a more practical nature than scientific. They focus on the whole syllabus and on common, rather than rare, conditions, e.g. pregnant women presenting with bleeding, vaginal discharge, vomiting or asking for advice after contact with someone with an infectious disease. It is expected that one should be able to make differentials, give advice and treat common conditions presenting in pregnancy.

When answering EMQs, one should be able to formulate an answer before going through the 10 options and then look to see if it fits with one of the answer options. This can save time and avoid confusion. Sometimes there can be two answers that are similar, so try to choose the most likely one. If you don't know the topic well, start eliminating the options one by one until you get a suitable option that seems like a close fit. Sometimes you may not know the answer, in which case, relax and take a logical approach to make an informed guess. Do not leave any questions unanswered as it can be difficult to return to them due to time constraints. This should allow you to gain marks rather than lose them as there is no negative marking. If you do have time at the end, it is worth going back and re-reading difficult questions to make sure that you have answered them correctly.

Always remember to read the question carefully as mistakes are made if you hurry. Often the question may seem familiar to you, but while similar, may in fact not be the exact same question that you have read before.

Multiple choice questions (MCQs)

MCQs assess a broader knowledge base and need more revision. One needs to know the facts in detail to be able to answer these questions correctly. *Get Through DRCOG* addresses this by giving explanations following each question-and-answer section, with appropriate references for further reading. You may refer to textbooks, read RCOG guidelines and websites or discuss with a senior colleague once you have identified any gaps in your knowledge.

Single best answer (SBA)

Five stems follow a single question and only one stem is either correct or wrong (true or false). The emphasis is on reading the question and answering carefully, as you should find it possible to answer each question correctly in most cases. Although you need some theoretical knowledge, some questions may be answered without any detailed knowledge.

Examination tips

In keeping with the current syllabus, the best time to sit for the DRCOG exam is while you are working in a department of obstetrics and gynaecology, as you can get hands-on practical experience in dealing with patients presenting with common problems, such as miscarriage, termination of pregnancy, antenatal care, management of labour and delivery, and consenting regarding obstetric and gynaecological procedures. By experiential learning you will have gathered the necessary knowledge regarding these topics through discussing various cases with senior colleagues or attending ward rounds, gynaecology outpatients, antenatal clinics or organized departmental teaching sessions. However, a theoretical base is important to ensure that you really understand why you are doing what you are doing whenever you undertake a particular task.

It is advisable to start planning and preparing at least 3 months before the examination as it can take a couple of weeks for revision to start gaining momentum. Also, the amount of information that you process can seem overwhelming. A key part of studying effectively is accessing information readily and quickly. Additionally, one has to tailor the study method according to the type of exam (e.g. essay writing, MCQs and EMQs). Therefore, organize yourself and take some time to explore what the exam is like, the type of questions you might encounter and the format of the exam. You can acquire detailed information from online examination websites, peers who have already taken the exam, the RCOG website and DRCOG courses. It is unlikely that a single website or textbook will adequately cover your entire exam objectives. So gather information and knowledge from at least two or three resources (e.g. websites, books and courses) for an improved understanding of how to pass the exam. Then make a list of common topics and themes repeated in the exam from the syllabus. From the beginning, highlight important topics or write down important points in a small notebook or make revision cards, so that you can revise the topics in a short period of time when the exam is approaching. Some people find it useful to discuss certain difficult topics with colleagues to help memorize facts or to improve overall understanding.

So plan ahead, make notes and revise common topics again. A week of study leave is ideal before the exam for revision purposes. Make sure that you are not working the day before the examination (it would be difficult to concentrate with the stress of work and lack of sleep). Be sure you know the time and place of your exam and plan to allow enough time to avoid the added pressure of running late.

Current trend for preparation

The current trend is for candidates to prepare for the examination using question and answer format by using DRCOG exam books and websites, as many of the themes tend to be repeated. *Get Through DRCOG* is an up-to-date exam book that covers all types of questions including EMQs, SBAs and MCQs for preparation before the exam. The questions follow the format of the DRCOG examination and are in keeping with the current syllabus. This book offers appropriate explanation and additional material following each question and answer so that you can develop your understanding of the common topics as well as practice your exam technique.

The following websites give information about the syllabus for the exam:

http://www.rcog.org.uk/guidelines
http://www.fsrh.org/
http://www.fsrh.org/pages/clinical_guidance.asp
http://guidance.nice.org.uk/CG/Published

Please visit the RCOG website for a further reading list for DRCOG exam.
Best of luck.

Rekha Wuntakal

ACKNOWLEDGEMENT

We would like to thank Ms Deepa Janga for her contribution to EMQ questions regarding antenatal care and gynaecological problems.

SBAs

Question 1

A 22-year-old Asian woman is admitted to the hospital with an incomplete miscarriage at 11 weeks' gestation. An ultrasound shows a 'snow storm' appearance. She passes grape-like vesicles through the vagina. She subsequently has a surgical evacuation of the uterus. The histology reveals a large mass with hydropic changes in all the placental villi and no fetal tissue. She is followed up with serum beta human chorionic gonadotrophin (βhCG) levels. There was an initial fall but it started to rise gradually (10,000 units/mL) at 3 months' follow up. Her CT scan chest, abdomen and pelvis are normal except localized thickened vascular area in the posterior wall of uterus. What is the likely diagnosis?

A. Gestational choriocarcinoma
B. Persistent trophoblastic disease
C. Non-invasive mole
D. Non-gestational choriocarcinoma
E. Placental site trophoblastic disease

Question 2

A 30-year-old woman presents to the early pregnancy unit with mild vaginal bleeding. An ultrasound is performed, which reports a complete molar pregnancy. What would be the parental origin and genetic complement of the complete molar pregnancy?

A. 2 paternal sets: diploid
B. 2 paternal sets: haploid
C. 1 paternal set: haploid
D. 2 paternal and 2 maternal sets: tetraploid
E. 1 maternal and 1 paternal set: diploid

Question 3

A 22-year-old Asian woman is admitted to the hospital with an incomplete miscarriage at 11 weeks' gestation. She subsequently has surgical evacuation of the uterus. The histology reveals a large mass with hydropic changes in all the placental villi with no fetal tissue. Which of the following is the most likely karyotype and parental chromosomal origin?

A. 46 XX, maternal
B. 46 XX, paternal
C. 46 XY, paternal
D. 69 XXY, paternal
E. 69 XXY, paternal and maternal

Question 4

A 22-year-old Asian woman is admitted to the hospital with an incomplete miscarriage at 11 weeks' gestation. She subsequently has surgical evacuation of the uterus. The histology reveals focal hydropic placental villi interspersed with normal villi and presence of fetal tissue. Which of the following is the most likely karyotype and parental chromosomal origin?

A. 46 XX, maternal
B. 46 XX, paternal
C. 46 XY, paternal
D. 69 XXY, paternal
E. 69 XXY, paternal and maternal

Question 5

Which one of the following statements is not true with respect to bacterial vaginosis (BV)?

A. Isolation of *Gardnerella vaginalis* on high vaginal swab culture is diagnostic of BV.
B. Vaginal pH is increased and is typically more than 4.5.
C. Presence of 'clue cells' on microscopy is diagnostic of bacterial vaginosis.
D. It is associated with preterm labour or miscarriage.
E. It is the commonest cause of abnormal vaginal discharge in women of reproductive age.

Question 6

In relation to the treatment of BV, which one of the following statements is true?

A. Routine treatment of male partners is recommended.
B. Vaginal douching is beneficial for symptomatic improvement.
C. Metronidazole is not safe during the first trimester of pregnancy.
D. Clindamycin 2% intravaginal cream is not effective.
E. Recurrent BV is difficult to manage as it can recur in up to 70% of females within 3 months of treatment.

Question 7

Which one of the following statements is false with respect to the risks of advanced maternal age?

A. Increased risk of pre-eclampsia
B. No increase or decrease in the stillbirth rate
C. Increased rate of instrumental delivery
D. Increased risk of gestational diabetes
E. Increased rate of caesarean section

Question 8

A 28-year-old para 1 woman with a dichorionic diamniotic (DCDA) twin pregnancy attends her antenatal appointment at 20 weeks' gestation. She is at risk of developing the following complications with the exception of which of the following?

A. Twin-to-twin transfusion syndrome
B. Pre-eclampsia
C. Postpartum haemorrhage
D. Fetal growth restriction
E. Preterm labour

Question 9

A 30-year-old para 2 woman with a BMI of 45 attends the antenatal clinic at 10 weeks' gestation. One of the following is incorrect with respect to the associated risks and counselling?

A. Increased risk of venous thromboembolism
B. Increased risk of pre-eclampsia
C. Folic acid 5 mg once a day supplementation
D. Vitamin D 100 micrograms daily supplementation during pregnancy
E. Increased risk of gestational diabetes

Question 10

A 38-year-old nulliparous woman with type 1 diabetes attends the antenatal clinic at 6 weeks' gestation. Which of the following is not an increased risk in her pregnancy?

A. Neural tube defects
B. Macrosomia
C. Congenital heart disease
D. Oligohydramnios
E. Pre-eclampsia

Question 11

With regard to the management of pregnant women with obesity (BMI ≥30), which one of the following statements is false?

A. Glucose tolerance test should be offered during pregnancy.
B. Folic acid 5 mg daily supplementation prior to and during pregnancy to minimize the risk of neural tube defects.
C. Induction of labour at 39 weeks is recommended.
D. They should have continuous electronic monitoring of the fetal heart during labour.
E. Active management of the third stage is recommended to minimize the risk of postpartum haemorrhage.

Question 12

Which one of the following drugs has no teratogenic effect?

A. Metronidazole
B. Sodium valproate
C. Warfarin
D. ACE inhibitors
E. Lithium

EMQs

OPTIONS FOR QUESTIONS 1–3

A. Refer routinely for colposcopy
B. Refer urgently for colposcopy
C. 5-year routine recall
D. 3-year routine recall
E. Repeat smear in 6 months
F. Repeat smear with an endocervical brush
G. Discharge to general practitioner
H. Annual smears for the next ten years
I. Discharge if three consecutive smears are normal
J. Repeat smear within 3 months
K. Perform high-risk HPV test
L. Perform low-risk HPV test

Instructions

Each clinical scenario described below tests knowledge about the interpretation of the cervical smear results. For each case, choose the single most appropriate course of action from the above list. Each option may be used once, more than once or not at all.

1. A 32-year-old woman with a normal smear 3 years ago has her current smear reported as a normal smear.
2. A 32-year-old woman with a normal smear 3 years ago has her current smear reported as glandular neoplasia.
3. A 32-year-old woman with a normal smear 3 years ago has her current smear reported as suspicious of possible invasion.

OPTIONS FOR QUESTIONS 4-6

A. Refer routinely for colposcopy
B. Refer urgently for colposcopy
C. 5-year routine recall
D. 3-year routine recall
E. Repeat smear in 6 months
F. Repeat smear with an endocervical brush
G. Discharge to general practitioner
H. Annual smears for the next ten years
 I. Discharge if three consecutive smears are normal
J. Repeat smear within 3 months
K. Perform high-risk HPV test
L. Perform low-risk HPV test

Instructions

Each clinical scenario described below tests knowledge about the interpretation of the cervical smear results. For each case, choose the single most appropriate course of action from the above list. Each option may be used once, more than once or not at all.

4. A 28-year-old woman with a normal smear 3 years ago has her current smear reported as mild dyskaryosis.
5. A 28-year-old woman with a normal smear 3 years ago has a current smear reported as borderline abnormality.
6. A 28-year-old woman with a normal smear 3 years ago has a current smear reported as normal smear with presence of actinomyces-like organisms.

OPTIONS FOR QUESTIONS 7–9

A. Refer routinely for colposcopy
B. Refer urgently for colposcopy
C. 5-year routine recall
D. 3-year routine recall
E. Repeat smear in 6 months
F. Repeat smear with an endocervical brush
G. Discharge to general practitioner
H. Annual smears for the next 10 years
I. Discharge if three consecutive smears are normal
J. Repeat smear within 3 months
K. Perform high-risk HPV test
L. Perform low-risk HPV test

Instructions

Each clinical scenario described below tests knowledge about the interpretation of the cervical smear results. For each case, choose the single most appropriate course of action from the above list. Each option may be used once, more than once or not at all.

7. A 30-year-old woman with a normal smear 3 years ago has a current smear reported as mild dyskaryosis. A high-risk HPV test on the liquid-based cytology (LBC) sample is positive.
8. A 30-year-old woman with a normal smear 3 years ago has a current smear reported as borderline dyskaryosis. The LBC sample is inadequate for HPV testing.
9. A 30-year-old woman with a normal smear 3 years ago has a current smear reported as mild dyskaryosis. The LBC sample is inadequate for HPV testing.

OPTIONS FOR QUESTIONS 10–12

A. Annual smears for the next 10 years
B. Discharge if three consecutive smears are normal
C. Discharge to general practitioner
D. 5-year routine recall
E. Perform smear test at 6 months, follow up
F. Perform smear test at 12 months, follow up (with or without colposcopy)
G. Repeat smear test in 6 months
H. Repeat smear with an endocervical brush
I. Refer routinely for colposcopy
J. Refer urgently for colposcopy
K. Repeat smear within 3 months
L. 3-year routine recall

Instructions

Each clinical scenario described below tests knowledge about the interpretation of the cervical smear results and treatment of smear abnormalities. For each case, choose the single most appropriate course of action from the above list. Each option may be used once, more than once or not at all.

10. A 33-year-old woman with a history of normal smear has a current smear reported as mild dyskaryosis. The LBC sample is positive for high risk HPV. She is therefore referred for routine colposcopy. Colposcopy reveals cervical intraepithelial neoplasia 1 (CIN 1). The woman prefers not to have excisional treatment.
11. A 33-year-old woman with a history of normal smear has a current smear reported as borderline smear. The LBC sample is positive for high risk HPV. She is therefore referred for routine colposcopy. Colposcopy reveals CIN 1. The woman prefers not to have excisional treatment.
12. A 33-year-old woman with a history of normal smear has a current smear reported as mild dyskaryosis. The LBC sample is positive for high risk HPV. She is therefore referred for routine colposcopy. Colposcopy reveals CIN 1. She has large loop excision of transformation zone (LLETZ) at the same setting for CIN 1.

OPTIONS FOR QUESTIONS 13–15

A. Missed miscarriage
B. Pregnancy of unknown location
C. Inevitable miscarriage
D. Threatened miscarriage
E. Ectopic pregnancy
F. Molar pregnancy
G. Complete miscarriage
H. Septic miscarriage
I. Recurrent miscarriage
J. Incomplete miscarriage

Instructions

For each clinical scenario below, choose the single most appropriate diagnosis from the options list. Each may be used once, more than once or not at all.

13. A 28-year-old woman presents at 8 weeks' gestation with abdominal pain and bleeding per vaginam. On speculum examination, there is no active bleeding and the cervix is closed. Ultrasound shows an intrauterine gestational sac with fetal pole and cardiac activity.

14. A 25-year-old nulliparous woman attends early pregnancy unit for a scan at 11 weeks' gestation after an episode of bleeding per vaginum. She denies any abdominal pain and admits that her nausea has resolved. Ultrasound shows an irregular intrauterine gestational sac measuring 32 mm with no fetal pole or yolk sac.

15. A 20-year-old woman presents with a history of vaginal bleeding and abdominal cramps at 10 weeks' gestation. Her pulse is 90 and BP is 140/90 mmHg. Ultrasound shows a 'snow storm appearance' with no fetal pole.

OPTIONS FOR QUESTIONS 16–18

A. *Bacterial vaginosis*
B. *Candida albicans*
C. *Chlamydia tracomatis*
D. *Clostridium botulinium*
E. *Haemophylus ducrei*
F. *Listeria monocytogenes*
G. *Molluscum contagiosum*
H. *Neisseria gonorrhoea*
I. *Treponema pallidum*
J. *Trichomonas vaginalis*
K. Yaws

Instructions

For each clinical scenarios described below, choose the most likely organism from the list above. Each answer can be used once, more than once or not at all.

16. A 19-year-old woman presents with non-specific vaginal discharge and lower abdominal pain. She had one partner 6 months ago and currently has a new partner who complains of dysuria and urethral discharge. Both attend the sexual health clinic for sexual health screening. Gram stain of urethral discharge from partner reveals gram-negative intracellular diplococci. What would be the causative organism in this case?

17. A 38-year-old woman presents with mild abdominal pain, diarrhoea and general malaise at 28 weeks' gestation. She complains of reduced fetal movements and rupture of membranes 6 hours ago. On examination the pad is wet and the appearance suggests meconium staining of the liquor. Speculum examination reveals a 2 cm dilated cervix and confirms preterm premature rupture of membranes. Abdominal examination reveals moderate contraction and a mildly tender abdomen. Ultrasound examination reveals an absent fetal heart beat and an intrauterine death of the fetus. What is the likely diagnosis in her case?

18. A 20-year-old woman presents to her GP with small lesions on her hand at 20 weeks' gestation. Examination reveals an umbilicated lesion on the inner thigh and vulva. Biopsy of the lesion and gram stain reveals eosinophilic inclusions in the epidermis. What is your likely diagnosis in her case?

MCQs

1. The risk factors for ectopic pregnancy include:
    A. Increased intake of alcohol
    B. Increased paternal age
    C. Previous pelvic inflammatory disease (PID)
    D. Previous pelvic surgery
    E. *In vitro* fertilization

2. Women with ectopic pregnancy can present with:
    A. Abdominal pain
    B. Vaginal bleeding
    C. Haematuria
    D. Collapse
    E. Headache

3. The following can be diagnostic features of ectopic pregnancy on transvaginal scan:
    A. Adnexal mass next to ovary
    B. Gestational sac within the uterine cavity
    C. Presence of corpus luteum in a single ovary
    D. Gestational sac in the abdominal cavity
    E. Distended bowel

4. Standard treatment modalities of ectopic pregnancy include:
    A. Surgical
    B. Medical
    C. Combined medical and surgical
    D. Bilateral salpingo-oophorectomy
    E. Hysterectomy

5. The diagnostic criteria for polycystic ovarian syndrome (PCOS) include:
    A. Anovulation
    B. Increased serum oestradiol levels
    C. Increased serum progesterone levels
    D. Increased serum luteinizing hormone levels
    E. Increased serum follicle-stimulating hormone levels

6. The hormonal and biochemical changes in PCOS include:
    A. Decreased LH:FSH ratio
    B. Hyperinsulinaemia
    C. Decreased serum testosterone levels
    D. Increased free-serum oestrogen levels
    E. Increased serum albumin levels

7. The following hormonal changes are seen in women with PCOS:
    A. Decrease in dehydroepiandrosterone sulphae (DHEAS)
    B. Increase in androstenedione
    C. Increase in serum oestradiol levels
    D. Decrease in serum oestrone levels
    E. Decrease in FSH levels

8. The various treatment modalities used in women with PCOS include:
   A. Weight loss
   B. Endometrial ablation
   C. Mirena IUS
   D. Cyproterone acetate
   E. Bilateral salpingo-oophorectomy

9. Chickenpox or varicella infection in pregnant women:
   A. Always causes fetal abnormalities in the fetus
   B. Can be transmitted to the fetus during 2nd trimester
   C. Can be transmitted to the fetus during 3rd trimester
   D. Is always transmitted to fetus antenatally
   E. Can be transmitted to the fetus during puerperium

10. The following are true with regard to chickenpox in pregnancy:
    A. The incubation period is less than 7 days.
    B. The infectious period starts after the onset of rash.
    C. The risk of spontaneous miscarriage is increased if chickenpox develops in the 1st trimester of pregnancy.
    D. The risk of premature delivery is increased if chickenpox develops in the 3rd trimester of pregnancy.
    E. The risk to the fetus is highest in the 3rd trimester of pregnancy.

11. Regarding chickenpox during pregnancy:
    A. Women who are exposed to chickenpox during pregnancy should have a blood test to check if they are immune to varicella.
    B. Women who are positive for IgG antibodies should be given varicella zoster immunoglobulin (VZIG).
    C. Women who are exposed to chickenpox during pregnancy should contact other pregnant woman to spread herd immunity.
    D. Women who develop chickenpox during pregnancy should receive VZIG.
    E. Women with chickenpox during pregnancy may develop varicella pneumonia.

12. Women with chickenpox during pregnancy should be advised to attend the emergency department if they develop the following symptoms:
    A. Rhinitis
    B. Neurological symptoms
    C. Haemorrhagic rash or bleeding
    D. Chickenpox rash on the body
    E. Diarrhoea

13. With regard to the Cervical Screening Programme guidelines in the UK:
    A. Cervical screening is offered to all women who are sexually active.
    B. Cervical screening is offered to women who are over 18 years and under 25 years of age.
    C. Cervical screening is offered to women 25–65 years of age.
    D. Cervical screening is offered every 3 years from the age of 25 years until the age of 49 years.
    E. Cervical screening is not offered to women with subtotal hysterectomy for benign conditions.

14. With regard to *Chlamydia trachomatis* infection:
    A. It is always sexually transmitted.
    B. It is the most common cause of non-gonococcal urethritis in men.
    C. Women with chlamydia infection can present with postcoital or intermenstrual bleeding.
    D. Only 40% of the women who have chlamydia infection are asymptomatic.
    E. Women with chlamydia infection can present with lower abdominal pain.

15. With regard to *Trichomonas vaginalis* infection:
    A. It is an intracellular bacteria.
    B. 90% of women are asymptomatic.
    C. Women may present with frothy vaginal discharge.
    D. It is a sexually transmitted infection.
    E. Metronidazole is the drug of choice used for its treatment.

16. The following organisms can cause pelvic inflammatory disease (PID):
    A. Streptococcus pneumonia
    B. Herpes simplex virus
    C. Hepatitis B virus
    D. Gonococcus
    E. Cytomegalovirus (CMV)

17. Women with PID can present with:
    A. Fever
    B. Vaginal discharge
    C. Lower abdominal pain
    D. Gastrointestinal bleeding
    E. Gastritis

18. Investigation may reveal the following in acute PID:
    A. Increased neutrophil count
    B. Increased white blood cell count
    C. Elevated erythrocyte sedimentation rate
    D. Decreased C-reactive protein
    E. Increased red blood cell count

19. The following drugs are used in the treatment of PID:
    A. Sulphadiazine
    B. Trimethoprim
    C. Ceftriaxone
    D. Oflaxacin
    E. Vancomycin

20. The following drugs are contraindicated in pregnancy:
    A. Penicillin
    B. Doxycycline
    C. Erythromycin
    D. Trimethoprim
    E. Low molecular weight heparin (enoxaparin)

21. The following factors increase the risk of cervical intraepithelial neoplasia (CIN):
    A. Immunosuppression
    B. Use of POP
    C. High socioeconomic status
    D. Smoking
    E. Late first pregnancy

22. Cervical screening fulfils the following WHO criteria for screening:
    A. It is an important health problem in the community.
    B. The natural history of the disease is not well known.
    C. There is a good screening test for diagnosis.
    D. There is a latent phase for detection and treatment of the condition early.
    E. Treatment at early stage is not beneficial for the condition.

23. With regard to treatment of CIN:
    A. The excisional treatment methods offer 100% cure rate.
    B. All ablative methods offer a cure rate of 70%.
    C. Only cryotherapy offers a cure rate of 100%.
    D. The cure following treatment is defined as normal smear at 5 years of follow up.
    E. The risk of recurrent CIN following treatment is around 5%.

24. The following infections can be diagnosed by wet-mount preparation of vaginal discharge:
    A. *Trichomonas vaginalis*
    B. *Bacterial vaginosis*
    C. *Vaginal candidosis*
    D. Beta-haemolytic streptococcus
    E. *Neisseria gonorrhoea*

25. With regard to hepatitis B antigens and antibodies:
    A. HBsAg appears in the blood soon after infection, before onset of acute illness.
    B. HBeAg disappears within 4–6 months after the start of clinical illness.
    C. HBsAg presence in mother indicates high risk of transmitting the disease to the fetus.
    D. Anti-Hbc disappears before HBsAg is gone.
    E. Anti-HBe presence in the mother indicates low risk of transmitting the disease to the fetus.

26. High-risk human papilloma viruses (HPVs):
    A. Can be detected in almost all cases of cervical cancer
    B. Can be associated with development of vulval cancers
    C. Can be associated with development of oropharyngeal cancers
    D. Are responsible for causing anogenital warts
    E. Are responsible for causing herpes infection

27. Human papilloma virus infection in the cervix:
    A. Needs treatment with antibiotics
    B. Needs treatment with anti-viral drugs in women under the age of 25
    C. Generally resolve spontaneously in most young women
    D. Is likely to persist when identified in older women when compared to younger women
    E. Stimulates the immune system and almost 90% of women will develop serum antibodies to HPV

28. Vulvar intraepithelial neoplasia (VIN):
    A. Incidence is increasing in young women
    B. Is unifocal disease in most young women
    C. Can arise in a background of lichen sclerosus
    D. Is more common in non-hair-bearing area of the vulva
    E. Can co-exist with cervical intraepithelial neoplasia (CIN) in 20–25% of cases

29. Women with VIN:
    A. Are asymptomatic in 80% of cases
    B. May present with pruritus
    C. May present with vulval lesion
    D. May present with dyspareunia
    E. May present with pelvic pain

30. With regard to VIN:
    A. Most young women with VIN have unifocal disease.
    B. Young women have a typical clinical presentation.
    C. In young women, VIN specifically arises in the labia majora.
    D. Women with VIN always need total vulvectomy to prevent recurrence of disease.
    E. Women with VIN should be offered colposcopy as it is associated with CIN.

31. Human papillomavirus (HPV):
    A. Is a RNA virus
    B. Is always transmitted by sexual contact
    C. Has predilection toward squamous epithelium
    D. Can cause pre-invasive lesions of the cervix
    E. Can cause benign genital warts

32. With regard to endometrial carcinoma:
    A. They occur in 50% of women with abnormal BRCA genes.
    B. They can be associated with HNPCC (hereditary nonpolyposis colorectal cancer) genes.
    C. They can be associated with non-dysjunction of genes.
    D. They can be easily diagnosed by performing routine cervical cytology.
    E. They have poorer prognosis stage-for-stage compared to ovarian cancers.

33. With regard to genetic gynaecological cancer syndromes:
    A. BRCA1 increases the risk of breast cancer by 80%.
    B. BRCA2 increases the risk of ovarian cancer by 20–30%.
    C. BRCA1 increases the risk of ovarian cancer by 100%.
    D. BRCA1 increases the risk of endometrial cancer by 80%.
    E. BRCA1 is associated with colorectal cancer.

34. With regard to hormone replacement therapy (HRT) in postmenopausal women:
    A. Oral HRT has more effect on coagulation than transdermal HRT.
    B. The incidence of venous thromboembolism (VTE) in premenopausal women is five times more than that of postmenopausal women.
    C. One should consider malignancy in the differential diagnosis in women who develop a denovo VTE after 50 years of age.
    D. If a postmenopausal woman is using transdermal HRT and develops VTE, she should be advised to continue HRT.
    E. All women should be screened for thrombophilia before initiation of HRT.

BASIC CLINICAL SKILLS – ANSWERS

SBAs

Answer 1: B

A molar pregnancy is a gestational trophoblastic disease that grows into a mass in the uterine cavity that has swollen or hydrophic chorionic villi (distention of the chorionic villi by fluid). The villi grow into grape-like clusters. On ultrasound scan this is described as 'honeycomb' or 'snow storm' appearance. Molar pregnancies are categorized as partial and complete moles. If untreated, these will almost always end in a spontaneous miscarriage. However, when diagnosed on ultrasound scan, women are offered a surgical evacuation of the uterus. Medical management is not recommended for molar pregnancy in view of theoretical risk of emboli of vesicles from the uterus.

Outcome following treatment of molar pregnancy

- Benign in more than 80%
- May develop into invasive mole or persistent trophoblastic disease in 10–15% ssses
- May develop into choriocarcinoma in 2–3% of cases
- During the next pregnancy, 98 out of 100 women will have a normal pregnancy and two women will have recurrent molar pregnancy.

Further reading

RCOG Green-top guideline No. 38. *Gestational trophoblastic disease*. 2010. Available at: www.rcog.org.uk/womens-health/clinical-guidance /management-gestational-trophoblastic-neoplasia-green-top-38

Answer 2: A

In most cases of complete molar pregnancy, all the genetic material is inherited from the father. In approximately 80% of these, possible mechanism is that a single sperm fertilizes an empty egg followed by a duplication of all the chromosomes. In rest of the cases (20%) an empty egg is fertilized by two sperms. In both cases the molar pregnancies are diploid.

Further reading

RCOG Green-top guideline No. 38. *Gestational trophoblastic disease*. 2010. Available at: www.rcog.org.uk/womens-health/clinical-guidance /management-gestational-trophoblastic-neoplasia-green-top-38

Hoffner L, Surti U. The genetics of gestational trophoblastic disease: a rare complication of pregnancy. *Cancer Genet* 2012; 205(3):63–77.

Answer 3: B

Complete moles are diploid and their chromosomes are purely paternal. In 90% of the complete moles, the karyotype is 46XX and in 10% it is 46XY.

Further reading

RCOG Green-top guideline No. 38. *Gestational trophoblastic disease*. 2010. Available at: www.rcog.org.uk/womens-health/clinical-guidance /management-gestational-trophoblastic-neoplasia-green-top-38

Hoffner L, Surti U. The genetics of gestational trophoblastic disease: a rare complication of pregnancy. *Cancer Genet* 2012; 205(3):63–77.

Answer 4: E

Partial moles are derived from both maternal and paternal chromosomes and are usually triploid (69XXY, 69XXX or 69XYY), with two sets of paternal chromosomes and one set of maternal chromosomes. Partial moles may result from two sperms fertilizing the ovum or from one sperm fertilizing the ovum and duplicating its chromosomes.

Further reading

RCOG Green-top guideline No. 38. *Gestational trophoblastic disease*. 2010. Available at: www.rcog.org.uk/womens-health/clinical-guidance /management-gestational-trophoblastic-neoplasia-green-top-38

Hoffner L, Surti U. The genetics of gestational trophoblastic disease: a rare complication of pregnancy. *Cancer Genet* 2012; 205(3):63–77.

Answer 5: A

BV is the commonest cause of abnormal discharge in the childbearing age group. It is not a sexually transmitted disease. It is caused by an overgrowth of mixed anaerobes replacing the dominant vaginal lactobacillus species, resulting in an increased vaginal pH to 4.5 to 7.0. Isolation of *Gardnerella vaginalis* on HVS culture is not diagnostic and is found in up to 30–40% of 'normal' women. BV usually presents with a profuse, homogenous, whitish grey, offensive smelling vaginal discharge. There is a characteristic fishy smell on adding 10% potassium hydroxide to the discharge and the presence of 'clue cells' on wet mount of the discharge is diagnostic of bacterial vaginosis. In pregnancy, BV is associated with late miscarriage, pre-term rupture of membranes, pre-term delivery and postpartum endometritis.

Further reading

Lazaro N. *Sexually Transmitted Infections in Primary Care*. 2nd ed. RCGP/BASHH. 2013. Available at: www.bashh.org/documents/Sexually%20Transmitted%20 Infections%20in%20Primary%20Care%202013.pdf

BASHH Clinical Effectiveness Group. *UK national guideline for the management of bacterial vaginosis 2012*. Available at: http://www.bashh.org/documents/4413 .pdf

Answer 6: E

Vaginal douching, bubble baths and antiseptics should be avoided as they alter the normal vaginal flora and increase the risk of BV. Routine screening and treatment of male partners is not advised as there is no reduction in relapse rates, though no evidence is available in treating female partners of lesbians with BV. Metronidazole is not teratogenic and is safe during the first trimester of pregnancy. Clindamycin 2% intravaginal cream daily for 7 days is a recommended treatment regimen, as is oral clindamycin 300 mg BD for 7 days. Treatment of recurrent BV is difficult to manage due to high recurrence rate after stopping treatment in up to 70% of women, even with metronidazole maintenance treatment.

Further reading

Lazaro N. *Sexually Transmitted Infections in Primary Care*. 2nd ed. RCGP/BASHH. 2013. Available at: www.bashh.org/documents/Sexually%20Transmitted%20 Infections%20in%20Primary%20Care%202013.pdf

BASHH Clinical Effectiveness Group. *UK national guideline for the management of bacterial vaginosis 2012*. Available at: http://www.bashh.org/documents/4413 .pdf

Answer 7: B

Advanced maternal age is associated with maternal and fetal complications like placental abruption, placenta previa, pre-eclampsia, gestational diabetes, malpresentation, low birth weight, pre-term and post-term delivery and postpartum haemorrhage. It is independently associated with an increase in antenatal and intrapartum stillbirth.

Further reading

RCOG SIP Opinion Paper No. 34. *Induction of labour at term in older mothers*. 2013. Available at: www.rcog.org.uk/files/rcog-corp/1.2.13%20SIP34%20IOL.pdf

Answer 8: A

Women with multiple pregnancies are at increased risk of miscarriage, anaemia, polyhydramnios, fetal growth restriction, pre-eclampsia, antepartum haemorrhage, placenta previa, pre-term labour and postpartum haemorrhage. Twin-to-twin transfusion syndrome is a specific complication in monochorionic monoamniotic twins due to vascular placental anastomosis, but not in DCDA twins.

Further reading

RCOG Green-top guideline No. 51. *Management of monochorionic twin pregnancy.* 2008. Available at: www.rcog.org.uk/womens-health/clinical-guidance /management-monochorionic-twin-pregnancy

Answer 9: D

Vitamin D 10 micrograms daily supplementation is recommended during pregnancy and while breastfeeding.

Further reading

CMACE/RCOG Joint Guideline. *Management of women with obesity in pregnancy.* 2010. Available at: www.rcog.org.uk/files/rcog-corp /CMACERCOGJointGuidelineManagementWomenObesityPregnancya.pdf

Answer 10: D

Women with pre-existing diabetes are at increased risk of congenital abnormalities like neural tube defects, congenital heart defects, skeletal abnormalities and sacral agenesis and unexplained intrauterine death at term. Babies tend to be macrosomic and associated with polyhydramnios. There is increased risk of operative delivery, birth trauma and shoulder dystocia. Postnatally, babies are at risk of hypoglycemia and neonatal jaundice.

Further reading

NICE clinical guideline No. 63. *Diabetes in pregnancy.* 2008. Available at: www.nice .org.uk/nicemedia/pdf/cg063guidance.pdf

Answer 11: C

Obesity alone is not an indication for induction of labour, as it carries the risk of failed induction and emergency caesarean section. Induction of labour should be reserved for specific obstetric and medical indications.

Further reading

CMACE/RCOG Joint Guideline. *Management of women with obesity in pregnancy*. 2010. Available at: www.rcog.org.uk/files/rcog-corp /CMACERCOGJointGuidelineManagementWomenObesityPregnancya.pdf

Answer 12: A

Metronidazole is safe in pregnancy; sodium valproate causes neural tube defects; warfarin causes skeletal and CNS defects and Dandy Walker syndrome; lithium causes Ebstein's anomaly, hypotonia, hyporeflexia and reduced suckling; and ACE inhibitors cause renal failure in neonates, decreased skull ossification and renal tubular dysgenesis.

Further reading

Collins S, Arulkumaran S, et al. *Oxford Handbook of Obstetrics & Gynaecology*. 3rd ed. Oxford: Oxford University Press; 2013.

EMQs

Answers 1–3

1. D

This woman had normal smear results in the past as well as present. She therefore needs 3-yearly routine recall.

2. B

Glandular neoplasia is often associated with cervical intraepithelial neoplasia (in 50% of cases) and an underlying malignancy (adenocarcinoma) in 40% of the cases. Therefore, one smear test reported as glandular neoplasia needs urgent referral to colposcopy and the woman needs to be seen in the clinic within 2 weeks of referral (target referral).

3. B

Possible invasion means suspected cancer. Therefore, urgent referral to colposcopy clinic is needed and the woman needs to be seen in the clinic within 2 weeks of referral (target referral).

Further reading

NHSCSP Publication No. 20. *Colposcopy and Programme Management. Guidelines for the NHS Cervical Screening Programme.* 2nd ed. 2010. Available at: www.bsccp.org.uk/colposcopy-resources/ colposcopy-and -programme-management-1

Answers 4–6

4. K

According to recent NHS cancer screening guidelines, women with borderline and mild dyskaryosis are triaged to have high-risk HPV test. If the high-risk HPV virus is positive then they are referred for colposcopy. If the colposcopy is normal, they then go on to have routine recall in 3 or 5 years' time depending on the screening age of patient. If the high-risk HPV test is negative then they go on to have routine recall in 3 years' or 5 years' time depending on the screening age of the patient.

Further reading

NHS Cancer Screening Programmes. *HPV Triage and Test of Cure Protocol: For Women Aged 25 to 64 Years.* 2010. Available at: www.cancerscreening.nhs.uk /cervical/hpv-triage-test-flowchart-v2.pdf

5. K

See preceding answer.

6. D

The presence of actinomyces in the cervical smear in an asymptomatic woman has no significance. It is not an indication for smear or repeat smear. Their presence is common in women with copper IUD. If the woman is symptomatic with pelvic pain and the smear shows actinomyces, she should be assessed and treated with antibiotics. If the coil is *in situ*, it should be removed.

Further reading

NHSCSP Publication No. 20. *Colposcopy and Programme Management. Guidelines for the NHS Cervical Screening Programme.* 2nd ed. 2010. Available at: www.bsccp.org.uk/colposcopy-resources /colposcopy-and-programme-management-1

Answers 7–9

7. **A**
8. **E**
9. **A**

HPV triage

Women referred due to borderline/mild cytology or normal cytology/HPV positive, who then have a satisfactory and negative colposcopy can be recalled in 3 years. If the cytology sample is unreliable or inadequate for the HPV test, refer mild dyskaryosis for colposcopy and recall borderline for 6-month repeat cytology. At repeat cytology perform HPV test. If HPV test is negative, return to routine recall; refer to colposcopy if HPV positive. Refer moderate or worse cytology for colposcopy.

Further reading

NHS Cancer Screening Programmes. *HPV Triage and Test of Cure Protocol: For Women Aged 25 to 64 years.* 2010. Available at: www.cancerscreening.nhs.uk /cervical/hpv-triage-test-flowchart-v2.pdf

Answers 10–12

10. **F**
11. **F**
12. **E**

HPV triage

- Untreated CIN 1 should be managed as per untreated CIN 1 following borderline/mild dyskaryosis.
- Follow up of 12-month cytology only should follow normal NHSCSP protocols.
- Women in annual follow up after treatment for CIN are eligible for the HPV test of cure at their next screening test.

Further reading

NHS Cancer Screening Programmes. *HPV Triage and Test of Cure Protocol: For women aged 25 to 64 years.* 2010. Available at: www.cancerscreening.nhs.uk /cervical/hpv-triage-test-flowchart-v2.pdf

Answers 13–15

13. D

In a case of threatened miscarriage, women present with bleeding ± abdominal pain, the cervical os is closed on examination and on ultrasound there is an intrauterine gestation sac with fetal pole and cardiac activity.

Further reading

Collins S, Arulkumaran S, et al. *Oxford Handbook of Obstetrics & Gynaecology.* 3rd ed. Oxford: Oxford University Press; 2013.

14. A

Missed miscarriage is diagnosed when a women presents with bleeding ± pain ± loss of pregnancy symptoms, cervical os is closed on speculum examination and on transvaginal ultrasound the mean gestational sac diameter is >25 mm with no visible fetal pole, or presence of a fetal pole >7 mm with no fetal heart activity.

Further reading

NICE clinical guideline 154. *Ectopic pregnancy and miscarriage: Diagnosis and initial management in early pregnancy of ectopic pregnancy and miscarriage.* 2012. Available at: www.nice.org.uk/nicemedia/live/14000/61854/61854.pdf

15. F

In molar pregnancy women tend to present with irregular vaginal bleeding during 1st trimester or with exaggerated pregnancy symptoms like hyperemesis, hyperthyroidism or early pre-eclampsia. On examination the uterus is usually large for dates and ultrasound features include characteristic 'snow storm appearance' of mixed echogenicity, representing hydropic villi and intrauterine haemorrhage.

Further reading

Collins S, Arulkumaran S, et al. *Oxford Handbook of Obstetrics & Gynaecology.* 3rd ed. Oxford: Oxford University Press; 2013.

Answers 16–18

16. H

Neisseria gonorrhoea is the second most common bacterial sexually transmitted infection in young men (20–24 years) and women (<20 years) in the UK. It is a gram-negative organism that can infect the mucous membrane of the pharynx, rectum, endocervix, urethra and conjunctivae. Men are usually symptomatic with a urethral discharge and dysuria. Women are symptomatic in less than 50% of cases. In women it can affect the pelvic organs, resulting in pelvic inflammatory disease.

Contact tracing is very important in managing sexually transmitted infections. Both patient and partner should be treated and advised to avoid sexual intercourse until they complete the course of antibiotics and are cleared of infection.

17. F

In this scenario, this woman has developed listeriosis.

- Listeriosis is caused by the bacterium *Listeria monocytogenes.*
- It is caused by eating contaminated food. The source of infection is usually water and soil, animal products such as meat and dairy products.
- It affects pregnant women, newborns and the immunosuppressed.
- Most often the symptoms go unnoticed. However, they may present with fever, muscle cramps and gastrointestinal symptoms.
- Pregnant women usually experience the above symptoms. Other people can present with CNS symptoms like headache and convulsions.
- Fetal risks during pregnancy include miscarriage, stillbirth and premature delivery and prematurity. The risks to the neonate include a serious life-threatening infection.
- One can prevent acquiring this infection by following certain safe practices. Pregnant women should be advised:
    - not to eat soft cheese such as feta, queso blanco, queso fresco, brie, camembert, panela, unless made with pasteurized milk; and
    - to wash fruits and vegetables before eating or cooking. Do not eat undercooked meat. Listeria is killed by pasteurization and cooking.
- The diagnosis is made following isolation of listeria from blood, cerebrospinal fluid, amniotic fluid or placenta during pregnancy. Gram staining (gram-positive motile bacterium) and culture can be used for their diagnosis. The culture will take 1–2 days and a negative culture does not generally rule out infection in the presence of symptoms. The role of serological tests and stool samples is limited.
- Listeriosis can be treated with antibiotics. Ampicillin is the drug of choice for its treatment. Gentamicin has been occasionally used in addition to ampicillin.

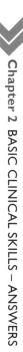

18. G

Molluscum contagiosum

- Pox virus
- Sexually transmitted disease
- More common in immunosuppressed-like HIV patients
- Incubation period: 3–12 weeks
- A self-limiting infection
- Spread by direct contact. Also by sharing towels and bathing sponge
- Lesions are usually single small pearly papules with umbilication
- Size of lesion is generally 2–5 mm
- Usually painless lesions
- Most lesions will regress spontaneously within 6–12 months
- Biopsy of the lesion will reveal molluscum bodies, which are viewed as eosinophilic inclusions in the epidermis
- May need treatment for cosmetic reasons
- Cryotherapy is effective. Laser therapy has also been used
- Podophyllotoxin 0.5% can be used but not recommended for pregnant women as may have teratogenic effect on the fetus
- Other agents include topical 5% potassium hydroxide, benzoyl peroxide, tretinoin, imiquimod. The last two cannot be used in pregnancy

Further reading

British Association for Sexual Health and HIV (BASHH). *National guideline on the diagnosis and treatment of gonorrhoea in adults.* 2005.

Centers for Disease Control and Prevention. *Clinical information: molluscum contagiosum.* 2011. Available at: www.cdc.gov/ncidod/dvrd/molluscum /clinical_overview.htm

MCQs

1A: False
1B: False
1C: True
1D: True
1E: True

The prevalence of ectopic pregnancy is 1–2%. It is the leading cause of maternal death in early pregnancy in the United Kingdom (0.2–0.35 maternal deaths/1000 ectopic pregnancies).

The risk factors for ectopic pregnancy include:

- Smoking
- Increased maternal age
- Assisted reproduction e.g. *in vitro* fertilization
- Previous PID
- Previous pelvic and abdominal surgeries including sterilization, recanalization of the fallopian tubes, salpingectomy, salpingostomy and appendisectomy
- More commonly seen in women with infertility
- Intrauterine copper device: it can increase the risk firstly by preventing the embryo from implanting in the uterine cavity and secondly by increasing the risk of developing PID
- Progoestogen-only pills
- Previous ectopic pregnancy

One should remember that almost 50% of women with ectopic pregnancy will not have prior risk factors.

Further reading

RCOG Green-top guideline No. 21. *Management of tubal pregnancy.* 2004.
    Available at: www.rcog.org.uk/womens-health/clinical-guidance
    /management-tubal-pregnancy-21-may-2004

2A: True
2B: True
2C: False
2D: True
2E: False

Women can present with different symptoms depending on the location of the ectopic pregnancy and the integrity of the tube.

The majority of the ectopic pregnancies (>90%) are in the fallopian tube. The most common site in the fallopian tube is the ampullary region. The other locations of ectopic pregnancy include cervix, ovary, caesarean section scar and, rarely, intra-abdominal.

History and symptoms

Women may present with symptoms or attend for a routine scan to the early pregnancy assessment unit. They usually present at 6–9 weeks' gestation. Late presentation at 12 weeks' gestation is seen in women with interstitial or cornual ectopic pregnancies. Women can present with abdominal pain or unilateral iliac fossa pain, vaginal bleeding, dizziness or a fainting episode. The typical symptoms of rupture include syncope, abdominal pain, shoulder tip pain, amenorrhoea, vomiting and diarrhoea and collapse (seen only in 20% of the patients). According to the Centre for Maternal and Child Enquiries (CEMACE) report on maternal deaths, women with ectopic pregnancy can present with atypical symptoms such as diarrhoea and vomiting. Therefore, one needs to be cautious in making a diagnosis of gastroenteritis rather than ectopic pregnancy when women present to the early pregnancy assessment unit with gastrointestinal symptoms. This may delay the diagnosis and lead to maternal death.

The clinical signs depend on the location of the ectopic pregnancy, integrity of the tube (rupture or unruptured ectopic) and the amount of blood in the peritoneal cavity. An ectopic pregnancy should be ruled out for all women presenting with abdominal pain to an early pregnancy assessment unit (EPAU) unless there are clear symptoms and signs of other conditions (e.g. UTI).

Unruptured ectopic pregnancy

Lower abdominal or unilateral iliac fossa tenderness is seen in women with an unruptured ectopic pregnancy. Some women may not have any clinical signs and are diagnosed only on a routine ultrasound scan.

Ruptured ectopic pregnancy

Abdominal examination will reveal tenderness, guarding and rigidity (signs of peritonism) if there is significant amount of blood in the peritoneal cavity. Pelvic examination will reveal severe adnexal tenderness and cervical excitation. Be gentle with pelvic examination as this may lead to rupture of an unruptured ectopic pregnancy.

Further reading

RCOG Green-top guideline No. 21. *Management of tubal pregnancy*. 2004. Available at: www.rcog.org.uk/womens-health/clinical-guidance /management-tubal-pregnancy-21-may-2004

Confidential Enquiries into Maternal and Child Health (CEMACH). *Why Mothers Die 2000–2002. The Sixth Report on the Confidential Enquiries into Maternal Deaths in the United Kingdom*. London: RCOG Press; 2004.

Confidential Enquiries into Maternal and Child Health (CEMACH). *Saving Mothers' Lives Report: Reviewing Maternal Deaths to Make Motherhood Safer: 2003–2005. The Seventh Report of the Confidential Enquiries into Maternal Deaths in the United Kingdom*. London: CEMACH; 2007.

Confidential Enquiries into Maternal and Child Health (CEMACH). Saving Mothers' Lives: Reviewing Maternal Deaths to Make Motherhood Safer: 2006–2008. The Eighth Report of the Confidential Enquiries into Maternal Deaths in the United Kingdom. *BJOG* 2011; 118 Suppl 1:1–203.

3A: True
3B: False
3C: False
3D: True
3E: False

Diagnosis is based on the history, examinations and investigations. In women with significant intraperitoneal bleeding, clinical signs are important to strongly suspect a diagnosis of ectopic pregnancy. However, if this is not the case, transvaginal scan (TVS) is the next step in making a diagnosis. The findings on TVS can be one of the following: (a) inhomogeneous echogenic mass in the adnexa (dirty snowball appearance); (b) a gestation sac with an echogenic ring all around (bagel sign); or (c) a gestational sac with a fetal pole or a yolk sac with or without cardiac activity.

Pregnancy of unknown location (PUL) is the terminology used when the uterine cavity is empty and there is no adnexal mass. In such women, one has to follow them carefully with symptoms assessment, serial beta human chorionic gonadotrophin (βhCG) serum levels and repeat transvaginal scan until a diagnosis is made or resolution of the condition occurs.

Further reading

Jurkovic D, Mavrelos D. Catch me if you scan: ultrasound diagnosis of ectopic pregnancy. *Ultrasound Obstet Gynecol.* 2007; 30(1):1–7.

4A: True
4B: True
4C: True
4D: False
4E: False

The management of ectopic pregnancy can be expectant, medical, surgical or a combination of the above.

Expectant management

Expectant management can be used in women who are asymptomatic or have minimal symptoms (abdominal pain), scan findings suggestive of small ectopic pregnancy or absence of free fluid or presence of minimal fluid in the pouch of Douglas and hormonal (βhCG) levels less than 1000 units/mL or if the diagnosis of PUL is made.

Medical management

The medical and social criteria for medical management (methotrexate use) include:

- Adnexal mass of <3.5 cm
- Serum βhCG levels <3000 units/mL (best results are obtained with serum βhCG levels <1500 units/mL. One can use this method with serum βhCG levels up to 5000 units/mL. However, non-resolution and intervention rates are high in women with high βhCG levels)
- Asymptomatic or minimal symptoms
- Absence of blood in the peritoneal cavity or very minimal fluid in the pouch of Douglas
- Absence of fetal cardiac activity
- Willing to follow up for the monitoring of symptoms and serial βhCG levels

Methotrexate is administered by a deep intramuscular injection of a single dose (50 mg/ m^2) in the management of ectopic pregnancy. If the response to methotrexate is suboptimal (serum βhCG levels showing a rise or suboptimal decline between 4–7 days of follow up), a second dose of methotrexate can be administered. If the patient does not respond to medical therapy or symptoms worsen and suggests of rupturing or ruptured ectopic, she would need surgical treatment.

Side effects of methotrexate

Side effects include stomatitis, nausea, vomiting, thrombocytopenia, hepatotoxicity and nephrotoxicity. Therefore, it is important to perform baseline full blood count, renal and liver function profiles before administering methotrexate.
Women should be clearly instructed that they should avoid getting pregnant for at least 3 months after the last injection of methotrexate in view of the risk of teratogenicity in the fetus.

Surgical management

The criteria for surgical management include:

- Woman unwilling for medical management or expectant management
- Woman wanting surgical management following discussion of the options
- Non-compliance for expectant or medical management
- Large adnexal mass
- βhCG levels more than 3000 units/mL
- Haemodynamic instability
- Collapse
- Presence of fetal cardiac activity
- Symptoms suggestive of ruptured ectopic

The Royal College of Obstetricians and Gynaecologists (RCOG) recommends salpingectomy when the contralateral tube is normal and salpingostomy when the contralateral tube is not healthy. The approach is usually laparoscopic in experienced hands unless there is haemodynamic instability needing urgent laparotomy or the surgeon is inexperienced. There is no difference with subsequent intrauterine pregnancy rates with either salpingostomy or salpingectomy. However, there is a risk of persistent trophoblastic tissue in the fallopian tube with salpingostomy. Serial βhCG follow up is therefore necessary following salpingostomy. Rise or suboptimal decline in the βhCG levels at follow up may necessitate further treatment in the form of medical therapy (methotrexate) or surgical treatment.

Further reading

RCOG Green-top guideline No. 21. *Management of tubal pregnancy.* 2004. Available at: www.rcog.org.uk/womens-health/clinical-guidance/management-tubal-pregnancy-21-may-2004

Lipscomb GH, Stovall TG, Ling FW. Primary care: non surgical treatment of ectopic pregnancy. *N Eng J Med.* 2000; 343: 1325–1329.

5A: **True**
5B: **False**
5C: **False**
5D: **False**
5E: **False**

European Society of Human Reproduction and Embryology (ESHRE) and American Society for Reproductive Medicine: proposed criteria for diagnosis of PCOS

PCOS is diagnosed if any two of the following are present:

- Ultrasound examination showing presence of polycystic ovaries (The Rotterdam consensus defines the polycystic ovary as having 12 or more follicles, measuring between 2 and 9 mm and/or an ovarian volume (OV) >10 cm^3)
- Biochemical or clinical hyperandrogenism
- Menstrual dysfunction with anovulation

Women have anovulatory cycles and therefore present with menstrual irregularity such as oligomenorrhoea or secondary amenorrheoa and rarely present with primary amenorrhoea. The other symptoms include acne and hirsutism without clinical signs of virilization. If symptoms or signs of virilization are present, one has to exclude late onset congenital adrenal hyperplasia and androgen-producing adrenal adenoma/tumours or ovarian tumours.
The other symptoms may include:

- Thinning of the scalp hair
- Weight gain
- Mental health problems

Women with PCOS are at risk of hypertension, type 2 diabetes and hypercholesterolaemia. So these women need long-term follow up and screening (at least yearly) for these conditions.

In PCOS, pelvic ultrasound scanning reveals polycystic ovaries (>12 follicles in each ovary and 10–11 mm size of each follicle). The follicles are generally placed at the periphery of the ovary giving a 'pearl necklace' appearance. Macroscopically the ovaries are enlarged and cut section shows an increase in the stroma of the ovary. Microscopically there is theca stromal cell hyperplasia surrounding arrested follicles.

Women with polycystic ovaries may not necessarily have PCOS. It may just be an incidental finding on the ultrasound scan seen in almost 25% of the women in reproductive age. These women are generally asymptomatic.

Criteria of the US National Institutes of Health: criteria for polycystic ovary syndrome and related disorders

Polycystic ovary syndrome

Presence of menstrual abnormalities and anovulation
Presence of clinical and/or biochemical hyperandrogenaemia
Absence of hyperprolactinaemia or thyroid disease
Absence of late-onset congenital adrenal hyperplasia
Absence of Cushing syndrome

Polycystic ovaries

Presence of polycystic ovaries on ultrasound examination
Absence of menstrual or cosmetic symptoms
Absence of biochemical hyperandrogenaemia

Idiopathic hirsutism

Presence of excess hair growth
Absence of biochemical hyperandrogenaemia

Further reading

RCOG Green-top guideline No. 33. *Long-term consequences of polycystic ovary syndrome.* 2007. Available at: www.rcog.org.uk/womens-health/clinical-guidance/long-term-consequences-polycystic-ovary-syndrome-green-top-33

European Society of Human Reproduction and Embryology (ESHRE). Available at: www.eshre.eu/

National Institutes of Health. *Evidence-Based Methodology Workshop on Polycystic Ovary Syndrome.* 2012. Available at: prevention.nih.gov/workshops/2012/pcos/docs/PCOS_Final_Statement.pdf

6A: False
6B: True
6C: False
6D: True
6E: False

Women with PCOS may present with any of the following symptoms:

- Amenorrhoea
- Oligomenorrhoea
- Infertility
- Hirsutism
- Combination of the above

LH:FSH ratio is increased in PCOS. Serum oestradiol levels are raised (PCOS is the only condition with raised serum oestrogen levels that is associated with anovulation) and as a result, there is no positive feedback on the hypothalamo-pituitary axis and, therefore, there is no 'LH surge'. This eventually leads to chronic anovulation. Also, high serum oestrogen levels (unopposed by progesterone) may increase the risk of developing endometrial hyperplasia and endometrial cancer. Therefore, it is important to ensure that these women have at least four periods a year (for endometrial shedding). This can be achieved by a withdrawal bleed using synthetic progestogens (e.g. Medroxyprogesterone acetate 10 mg once daily for 10 days). The other option is Mirena IUS for these women. This provides both protection against endometrial hyperplasia (and endometrial cancer) and contraception.

PCOS is associated with hyperinsulinaemia and peripheral insulin resistance which may be aggravated by the presence of obesity. The increase in serum LH from the anterior pituitary will also result in theca cell hyperplasia and an increase in the ovarian stroma leading to increase in the production of androgens (testosterone and androstenedione). This contributes to the symptoms of hyperandrogenism (acne and hirsutism). Insulin-like growth factor-1 (IGF-1) may have a similar effect on the ovarian function.

Hyperinsulinemia may also lead to dyslipidemia and elevated levels of plasminogen activator inhibitor 1 (PAI-1) in these women. The latter is a risk factor for intravascular thrombosis. These women are also at risk of developing hypertension, type 2 diabetes mellitus, coronary artery disease and cerebrovascular accidents. Therefore, women with PCOS should be thoroughly counselled regarding short-term as well as long-term risks of PCOS and the need for annual screening of hypertension and diabetes. Obese women should be advised to lose weight.

Some women may have skin changes called acanthosis nigricans (which is thought to be due to insulin resistance). It is a diffuse hyperpigmented velvety thickening of the skin generally seen in the axilla, nape of the neck and beneath the breasts.

Further reading

RCOG Green-top guideline No. 33. *Long-term consequences of polycystic ovary syndrome.* 2007. Available at: www.rcog.org.uk/womens-health/clinical-guidance/long-term-consequences-polycystic-ovary-syndrome-green-top-33

7A: False
7B: True
7C: False
7D: False
7E: True

Hormonal and biochemical changes seen in PCOS include:

- Increase in serum insulin levels and insulin resistance
- Impaired glucose tolerance
- Increase in serum LH levels (not necessary for diagnosis of PCOS)
- Normal or decrease in serum FSH levels
- Decrease in sex hormone binding levels (SHBG)
- Decrease in serum oestradiol levels
- Increase in serum oestrone (due to peripheral conversion of androgen to oestrogens by aromatization in adipose tissue)
- Increase in free oestrogen levels
- Increase in free androgen levels (androgen mainly bind to SHBG, which is decreased in PCOS and therefore free androgen levels are increased)
- Increase in serum testosterone levels
- Increase in androstenedione levels
- Increase in DHEAS levels
- Increase in insulin-like growth factor 1 (IGF-1) levels
- Plasminogen activator inhibitor 1 (PAI-1)
- Increase in cholesterol levels
- Increase in very low density lipoproteins (VLDL) levels
- Increase in low density lipoproteins (LDL) levels
- Increase in serum triglycerides
- Decrease in high-density lipoproteins (HDL) levels

Further reading

RCOG Green-top guideline No. 33. *Long-term consequences of polycystic ovary syndrome.* 2007. Available at: www.rcog.org.uk/womens-health/clinical-guidance/long-term-consequences-polycystic-ovary-syndrome-green-top-33

8A: True
8B: False
8C: True
8D: True
8E: False

The treatment of women with PCOS depends on the symptoms at presentation.

- Obesity and psychological impact: 50% of the women with PCOS are obese. The first step in the management is counselling on weight loss. This can be achieved either by regular exercise, weight-losing drugs (Orlistat, Rimonabant and Sibutramine) or bariatric surgery. Psychological counselling is important as these women often have low self esteem.
- Menstrual disturbances: 5–10% loss of body weight will normally restore the menstrual period. If menstrual irregularity is the main issue, woman can be advised to take combined oral contraceptive pills (also provides contraception) or can be given medroxyprogesterone acetate 10 mg once daily for 10 days to elicit withdrawal bleed.
- Hirsuitism and acne: physical methods such as waxing, shaving and electrolysis can be advised for increase in facial and body hair. The medical treatment for hirsutism includes anti-androgen drug therapy with cyproterone acetate and spironolactone. If the woman has acne and fluid retention problems premenstrually, the use of drosperinone (yasmin) may be considered (also provide contraception). The other drugs used in the treatment of hirsutism include flutamide, ketaconazole, finsateride, and depilatory local creams.
- Infertility: women presenting with infertility can be treated with clomiphene citrate or gonadotrophins (as these women have anovulatory cycles). Women resistant to clomiphene citrate may need ovarian drilling (surgical treatment). However, one still needs to emphasize weight optimization with these women.
- Pregnancy: women with PCOS who get pregnant are at increased risk of early miscarriage. They are also at risk of developing gestational diabetes and hypertension. It is important to monitor for these conditions and treat as necessary.

Further reading

RCOG Green-top guideline No. 33. *Long-term consequences of polycystic ovary syndrome.* 2007. Available at: www.rcog.org.uk /womens-health/clinical-guidance/ long-term -consequences-polycystic-ovary-syndrome-green-top-33

9A: False
9B: True
9C: True
9D: False
9E: True

Varicella zoster (VZ) virus is an infectious disease transmitted by close contact, respiratory droplets or by traplacental route to the fetus. Fetal transmission of the virus can occur in any trimester of pregnancy but the effects of infection (2% risk of congenital fetal varicella syndrome) are mainly seen before 20 weeks' gestation. The abnormalities (damage to eyes, scarring of skin, limb hypoplasia) in the fetus can be evident on ultrasound scan 4 to 5 weeks after the maternal infection. Therefore, the recommendation is to offer a detailed fetal scan 5 weeks following maternal infection to detect any fetal abnormalities. This should be performed by a fetal medicine specialist.

If the virus is transmitted at a later gestation, it generally remains dormant in the fetus and can present as shingles later in life.

There is significant risk to the newborn if maternal infection occurs at term. If the onset of maternal symptoms develops in the week following delivery, the neonate should be given Varicella zoster immunoglobulin (VZIG) and monitored for the next 4 weeks after the onset of maternal rash. If the newborn baby comes in contact with somebody who has chickenpox during the first 7 days of their life, no intervention is required, if the mother is immune. However, if the mother is not immune, the neonate should be given VZIG.

Further reading

RCOG Green-top guideline No. 13. *Chickenpox in pregnancy.* September 2007. Available at: www.rcog.org.uk/womens-health/clinical-guidance /chickenpox-pregnancy-green-top-13

10A: False
10B: False
10C: False
10D: False
10E: False

The incubation period is 7–21 days. The patients usually present with flu-like symptoms and rash. The infectiousness starts 48 hours before onset of rash until vesicles have crusted. If women develop chickenpox during pregnancy it carries 2% risk of congenital fetal varicella syndrome before 20 weeks' gestation. For the mother, it increases the morbidity as well as the mortality by causing life-threatening pneumonia (10% mortality), hepatitis and encephalitis (often chickenpox in early pregnancy is more dangerous to the fetus and in later pregnancy is more fatal for the mother).

Women should be advised that the risk of spontaneous miscarriage does not seem to be increased if chickenpox occurs in the first trimester.

The risk of congenital fetal varicella syndrome in the third trimester is negligible. There are no cases reported after 28 weeks' gestation.

Paediatricians should be made aware of the maternal condition, so that they follow up the neonate and infant for ophthalmic examination and review of symptoms.

Further reading

RCOG Green-top guideline No. 13. *Chickenpox in pregnancy.* September 2007. Available at: www.rcog.org.uk/womens-health/clinical-guidance /chickenpox-pregnancy-green-top-13

11A: True – Most women (>90%) in the UK are immune to VZV infection. Therefore, a blood test should be performed to check for IgG antibody. If positive for IgG antibody, it indicates immunity. If this is the case, the woman can be reassured.
11B: False
11C: False
11D: False
11E: True

Pregnant women should be advised to contact their GP if they come in contact with children with chickenpox or develop a rash on their body. They should also avoid contact with other pregnant women and neonates.

If a woman comes in contact with a child who has chickenpox, their serum should be checked for varicella IgG antibodies. If positive for antibodies, they should then be reassured and require no further treatment. If negative for IgG antibodies, then she is at risk of developing chickenpox. She should receive VZIG if she presents within 10 days of exposure. VZIG has no therapeutic benefit once chickenpox has developed.

Oral acyclovir should be prescribed for pregnant women with chickenpox if they present within 24 hours of the onset of the rash and if the gestational age is >20 weeks. It reduces the duration of disease and severity of symptoms.

Further reading

RCOG Green-top guideline No. 13. *Chickenpox in pregnancy.* September 2007. Available at: www.rcog.org.uk/womens-health/clinical-guidance /chickenpox-pregnancy-green-top-13

Tunbridge AJ, Breuer J, Jeffery KJM, on behalf of the British Infection Society. Chickenpox in adults – clinical management. *J Infect.* 2008; 57, 95–102.

12A: False
12B: True
12C: True
12D: False
12E: False

Women with severe symptoms (chest, neurological or haemorrhagic rash or bleeding) may need hospitalization in intensive care unit (ICU). They should be isolated from other pregnant women, babies and non-immune staff.

Further reading

RCOG Green-top guideline No. 13. *Chickenpox in pregnancy.* September 2007. Available at: www.rcog.org.uk/womens-health/clinical-guidance /chickenpox-pregnancy-green-top-13

13A: False
13B: False
13C: True
13D: True
13E: False

Cervical screening is a test to identify and treat early abnormalities (precancer) that, if left untreated, may lead to cancer. National Health Service Cervical Screening Programme (NHSCSP) guidelines in the UK recommend starting cervical screening at the age of 25 years. Women will have cervical smears every 3 years until the age of 49 years and then every 5 years until the age of 65. For women who have undergone subtotal hysterectomy for benign conditions, the cervix is retained; therefore, these women should continue to have cervical smears until the age of 65. Women under 25 years of age are not offered screening as the incidence of cervical cancer is rare in this age group and, at the same time, there is a high rate of human papillomavirus (HPV) infection, which is usually self limiting.

Further reading

NHSCSP Publication No. 20. *Colposcopy and Programme Management. Guidelines for the NHS Cervical Screening Programme.* 2nd ed. 2010. Available at: www.bsccp.org.uk/colposcopy-resources/colposcopy-and -programme-management-1

14A: False – Neonates acquire this infection during childbirth and mainly manifest as conjunctivitis.
14B: True
14C: True
14D: False
14E: True

Chlamydia is the most common treatable sexually transmitted disease in the UK.

Its prevalence in the UK is around 10%. The causative organism for chlamydia is gram-negative intracellular bacterium that infects columnar and transitional epithelium.

The risk factors for chlamydia include age below 25 years, more than one partner within a year, new partner, lack of barrier contraception, poor socioeconomic status, infection with another sexually transmitted disease and women undergoing termination of pregnancy. Women can present with abdominal pain, abnormal cervical or mucopurulent vaginal discharge, postcoital or intermenstrual bleeding. However, most men (>50%) and women (80%) with this infection are asymptomatic.

Chlamydia trachomatis (symptoms and sequelae)

Chlamydia trachomatis (an intracellular pathogen) is the causative organism. The incubation period is 1–3 weeks. Only certain strains of the organism cause pelvic infection. Serovars A, B, Ba or C are associated with trachoma (a major cause for blindness worldwide). Serovars L1, L2, L3 are associated with lymphogranuloma venerium. Serovars D–K cause non-specific urethritis and epididymitis in men; and perihepatitis, cervicitis, urethritis, endometritis, salpingitis (infection of upper genital tract, leading to pelvic inflammatory disease [PID]) in women. It can cause Reiter's syndrome in both men and women (conjunctivitis, proctitis, urethritis and reactive seronegative arthritis). The long-term sequelae include tubal damage, PID, chronic pelvic pain, Fitz-Hugh–Curtis syndrome, infertility and ectopic pregnancy. It is also associated with increased rates of transmission of HIV infection.

Investigations

Endocervical or urethral swabs (first sample of urine in men) are collected for culture and nucleic acid amplification test. It is highly sensitive and specific.

Treatment

Chlamydia infection is highly sensitive to doxycycline and the erythromycin group of drugs. Doxycycline is contraindicated during pregnancy. Erythromycin is recommended during pregnancy.

Contact tracing is important to treat the chain of people involved in transmitting the infection. One should advise to avoid sexual intercourse or use barrier contraception until the infection is treated and a test of cure is performed.

Neonatal transmission

- Conjunctivitis (incubation period is 1–3 weeks)
- Pneumonia
- Asymptomatic carriage

Further Reading

NHS and HPA. *National Chlamydia Screening Programme Standards*. 6th ed. 2012. Available at: www.chlamydiascreening.nhs.uk/ps/resources/core-requirements/NCSP%20Standards%206th%20Edition_October%202012.pdf

15A: False
15B: False
15C: True
15D: True
15E: True

Trachomonas vaginalis is a flagellated protozoan. It causes trichomoniasis, which is a sexually transmitted infection. Women usually present with vaginal discharge (70%) or frothy yellowish vaginal discharge (<30%), vulval itching and dysuria (urethral infection is seen in 90% of cases). Some women may present with lower abdominal pain and a few others may show signs of vaginitis and vulvitis. However, 50% of women may be asymptomatic. Contact bleeding from the cervix and strawberry appearance of the cervix (2% of cases) can be seen on speculum examination. A wet mount on microscopy will reveal a flagellated organism. A high vaginal swab for culture will be diagnostic in most cases (95%). The drug of choice for its treatment is metronidazole (single dose of 2 gm or 400 mg twice daily for 7 days) and this can be used in all trimesters of pregnancy. However, the use of a higher dose regimen should be avoided during pregnancy. Screening for other sexually transmitted diseases (STIs) should be offered and sexual partners should be treated. They should also be advised abstinence until treatment is completed. Trichomonas in young children raises the possibility of sexual contact and one should not rule out sexual abuse.

Further reading

Collins S, Arulkumaran S, et al. *Oxford Handbook of Obstetrics & Gynaecology*. 3rd ed. Oxford: Oxford University Press; 2013.

16A: False – It is responsible for causing meningitis, pneumonia and septic arthritis.
16B: True
16C: False
16D: True
16E: True – CMV is a less common cause of PID.

PID comprises a spectrum of inflammatory disorders of the upper genital tract, including salpingitis, endometritis, tubo-ovarian abscess, pelvic peritonitis or a combination of these. Many women with PID may not have symptoms or may have minimal symptoms. This may delay the diagnosis and contribute to inflammatory damage of the upper genital tract. The exact prevalence of the disease is difficult to ascertain because of its asymptomatic nature in most women.

The following organisms have been implicated in causing PID (some more than others).

Most common causes of PID

- *Chlamydia trachomatis*
- *Neisseria gonorrhoeae*

Less common causes of PID

- Anaerobes
- *Gardnerella vaginalis*
- *Haemophilus influenza*
- Enteric gram-negative rods
- *Streptococcus agalactiae*
- Cytomegalovirus
- *Mycoplasma hominis*
- *Ureaplasma urealyticum*
- *Mycoplasma genitalium*
- Herpes simplex type 2
- *Actinomyces israelii*

Long-term sequelae of PID

- Chronic pelvic pain
- Chronic PID
- Ectopic pregnancy
- Infertility

Further reading

Collins S, Arulkumaran S, et al. *Oxford Handbook of Obstetrics & Gynaecology*. 3rd ed. Oxford: Oxford University Press; 2013.

17A: True
17B: True – Women present with abnormal cervical or mucopurulent vaginal discharge. They may also present with dyspareunia because of the pelvic inflammation and adhesion caused by PID.
17C: True – Signs: abdominal and pelvic examination may reveal one or more of the following: (1) adnexal tenderness; (2) uterine tenderness; (3) unilateral or bilateral iliac fossa tenderness or lower abdominal tenderness.
17D: False – Women with PID present with intermenstrual or postcoital bleeding. Young women presenting with these symptoms should be at least screened for three things: (1) chlamydia infection; (2) to rule out local cervical causes for bleeding e.g. polyp or ectropion or cancer; (3) use of contraceptive pills, especially progestogen-only pills or depot medroxyprogesterone acetate or implananon or mirena IUS.
17E: False

Further reading

Collins S, Arulkumaran S, et al. *Oxford Handbook of Obstetrics & Gynaecology*. 3rd ed. Oxford: Oxford University Press; 2013.

18A: True
18B: True
18C: True
18D: False – C-reactive protein is raised.
18E: False

Further reading

Centers for Disease Control and Prevention. *Sexually transmitted diseases treatment guidelines 2010 – Pelvic inflammatory disease*. 2010. Available at: www.cdc.gov /std/treatment/2010/pid.htm

Collins S, Arulkumaran S, et al. *Oxford Handbook of Obstetrics & Gynaecology*. 3rd ed. Oxford: Oxford University Press; 2013.

19A: False
19B: False – Used for treating acute urinary tract infection (UTI) and prophylaxis for recurrent UTI

19C: True – Effective against *Neisseria gonorrhoeae*
19D: True
19E: False

The various drugs that can be used in the treatment of PID include (Centers for Disease Control and Prevention)

- Ceftriaxone
- Doxycycline
- Metronidazole
- Cefoxitin
- Cefotetan
- Clindamycin
- Gentamycin
- Ampicillin/Sulbactam
- Azithromycin
- Oflaxacin

The drugs commonly used for treatment of PID in UK include (depending on the local protocol)

- Doxycycline
- Ceftriaxone
- Metronidazole
- Ofloxacin

Further reading

Centers for Disease Control and Prevention. *Sexually transmitted diseases treatment guidelines 2010 – Pelvic inflammatory disease.* 2010. Available at: www.cdc.gov /std/treatment/2010/pid.htm

Collins S, Arulkumaran S, et al. *Oxford Handbook of Obstetrics & Gynaecology.* 3rd ed. Oxford: Oxford University Press; 2013.

20A: False – Penicillins and cephalosporins are used as first-line drugs for the treatment of common conditions during pregnancy e.g. urinary tract infection (UTI), pharyngitis. They are safe to be used in all trimesters of pregnancy and during breastfeeding.
20B: True – The tetracycline group of drugs are contraindicated as they can damage the enamel of the teeth and also cause discolouration of the teeth.
20C: False – Erythromycin is safe both during pregnancy and breastfeeding. It is used as a first line in women who are allergic to penicillin.
20D: True – Trimethoprim is contraindicated during the 1st trimester of pregnancy due to its teratogenic effects (folate antagonist). It can be used in the 2nd and 3rd trimester of pregnancy for the treatment of UTI. It can also be used for prophylaxis in women with recurrent UTI (2 or more) during pregnancy. It is excreted in the breast milk but is not harmful to the baby.

20E: False – Enoxaparin does not cross the placenta. It can be safely used both during pregnancy and breastfeeding. It is used for both prophylaxis and treatment of deep vein thrombosis (DVT) and pulmonary embolism (PE) during pregnancy.

On the other hand, warfarin is contraindicated in pregnancy as there is an increased risk of congenital abnormalities and intracranial haemorrhage with its use. If the patient is taking warfarin prior to pregnancy for prophylaxis or treatment of DVT or PE, it would need to be changed into LMWH, which can be given subcutaneously. This should preferably be done before conception to reduce the risk of teratogenicity or as soon as the diagnosis of pregnancy is made.

Further reading

BNF 2013–14: British National Formulary. Vol. 66. London: Pharmaceutical Press and BMJ Group; 2013– 2014.

21A: True
21B: False
21C: False
21D: True
21E: False

The risk factors for development of cervical intraepithelial neoplasia include

- High risk HPV infection
- Persistence of HPV infection
- Early age at sexual intercourse
- Multiple sexual partners (male or female)
- Cigarette smoking
- Low socioeconomic status
- Increases with increasing number of pregnancies

The risk decreases to some extent with the use of condoms and late first pregnancy.

Further reading

RCOG risk factors tutorial. *Summary of risk factors leading to the development of genital tract intraepithelial neoplasia.* Available at: www.rcog.org.uk /stratog/page/summary-risk-factors-leading-development-genital-tract -intraepithelial-neoplasia

22A: True
22B: False
22C: True
22D: True
22E: False

WHO criteria for screening (1968)

Wilson-Jungner criteria for appraising the validity of a screening programme

- The condition must be an important public health problem.
- The natural history of the disease should be well known or understood.
- There should be a latent phase of the disease when it can be detected.
- Presence of a suitable and acceptable screening test.
- The test should be simple, safe, reliable and validated.
- Intervals for repeating test should be determined.
- Presence of an acceptable intervention for the patient with the condition.
- Presence of facilities for diagnosis and treatment of the condition.
- Treatment at an early stage should be of more benefit than at a later stage.
- The primary prevention interventions should be cost effective.
- Both physical and psychological risks should be less than the benefits.
- Case findings should not be a one-off process but a continuous process.
- Adequate health service provision should be made for extra clinical workload.

Further reading

RCOG reflective task tutorial. *Pre-invasive disease of the lower genital tract.* Available at: www.rcog.org.uk/stratog/page/reflective-task-3

gp-training.net. *Screening criteria.* Available at: www.gp-training.net/training/tutorials/management/audit/screen.htm

23A: False – The cure rate following excisional treatment of CIN is 95%.
23B: False – Ablative methods offer a cure rate of 90–95% except cryotherapy.
23C: False – Cryotherapy offers a cure rate of 85% and this has been attributed to inadequate depth of tissue destruction.
23D: False – The cure following treatment is defined as normal smear at 6-month follow up.
23E: True – The risk of recurrent CIN following treatment is around 5%.

Further reading

RCOG risk factors tutorial. *CIN treatment.* Available at: www.rcog.org.uk/stratog/page/available-techniques-treating-cin

24A: True – Wet mount reveals motile protozoa.
24B: True – Wet mount shows clue cells.
24C: True – Wet mount shows hyphae and spores.
24D: False – Beta-haemolytic streptococcus needs gram staining and culture.
24E: False – *Neisseria gonorrhoea* can be seen as kidney-shaped intracellular diplococci on gram staining.

Further reading

Collins S, Arulkumaran S, et al. *Oxford Handbook of Obstetrics & Gynaecology.* 3rd ed. Oxford: Oxford University Press; 2013.

Lazaro N. *Sexually Transmitted Infections in Primary Care.* 2nd ed. RCGP/BASHH. 2013. Available at: www.bashh.org/documents/Sexually%20Transmitted%20 Infections%20in%20Primary%20Care%202013.pdf

25A: True
25B: False – HBeAg appears in acute phase and disappears before HBsAg is gone. Its presence indicates higher risk of transmitting the disease to fetus from mother.
25C: False – It appears in the beginning of the acute illness and is seen during the window period.
25D: False
25E: True

Further reading

Collins S, Arulkumaran S, et al. *Oxford Handbook of Obstetrics & Gynaecology.* 3rd ed. Oxford: Oxford University Press; 2013.

26A: True – More than 100 types of HPV virus have been described and out of these the most common genotypes include HPV 16, 18, 31 and 33. In more than 70% of the cases of cervical cancers HPV 16 and 18 have been implicated as causative viruses
26B: True
26C: True
26D: False – Low-risk HPV types 6 and 11 cause ano-genital warts. Routine HPV testing is not recommended to diagnose genital warts. Clinical examination is sufficient to diagnose genital warts. Cervical lesions may need colposcopy if there is suspicion of dysplasia or malignancy.
26E: False

Further reading

Collins S, Arulkumaran S, et al. *Oxford Handbook of Obstetrics & Gynaecology.* 3rd ed. Oxford: Oxford University Press; 2013.

27A: False – HPV infections are not treated by antibiotics.
27B: False – Asymptomatic HPV infections do not require any treatment.
27C: True – Transient HPV infection is more common in women less than 25 years of age. These women are generally asymptomatic and the infection clears spontaneously within 2 years. Low-grade abnormalities are also common in this age group, which would resolve spontaneously. Therefore, screening these women with cervical cytology would create greater anxiety, colposcopic examinations, treatments and its consequences. The incidence of cervical cancer in women under 25 years is low and screening these women has not been shown to reduce the incidence of cervical cancer. In view of the above reasons cervical screening is not recommend in women under the age of 25. Women under 25 years who are concerned about their sexual health or risk of developing cervical cancer should contact their GP or genitourinary medical clinic.

27D: True – Older women are generally less likely to clear HPV than younger women.
27E: False – Only 50–60% of women will develop antibodies following HPV infection.

Further reading

Guidelines for the NHS Cervical Screening Programme. 2nd ed. *Colposcopy and Programme Management*. NHSCSP Publication No. 20. 2010.

Collins S, Arulkumaran S, et al. *Oxford Handbook of Obstetrics & Gynaecology*. 3rd ed. Oxford: Oxford University Press; 2013.

28A: True
28B: False – VIN is multifocal in most young women.
28C: True – Cellular atypia is seen in >25% of patients with lichen sclerosis (usually associated with differentiated VIN). Women with lichen sclerosis have a 3–5% risk of developing vulval cancer.
28D: True – Labia minora is more commonly involved in VIN.
28E: True – Since it can co-exist with CIN, colposcopic examination of the cervix should be performed in these women.

Further reading

RCOG Green-top guideline No. 58. *The management of vulval skin disorders*. 2011. Available at: www.gp-training.net/training/tutorials/management/audit/screen.htm

Collins S, Arulkumaran S, et al. *Oxford Handbook of Obstetrics & Gynaecology*. 3rd ed. Oxford: Oxford University Press; 2013.

29A: False – Around 50% of women with VIN are asymptomatic.
29B: True
29C: True – Vulval examinations can reveal erythematous areas, leukoplakic patches, ulcerated and pigmented areas.
29D: True
29E: False

VIN can be differentiated or warty and basaloid, which is the usual type. Differentiated VIN may be unifocal and common in postmenopausal women. It is associated with lichen sclerosus and is a high risk for developing into a squamous cell carcinoma. It is not graded and is not associated with CIN.

The usual or warty type can be multifocal and present in premenopausal women. Although associated with HPV, smoking and immunodeficiency, it is associated with a low risk of malignancy (squamous cell carcinoma). It is graded like CIN.

Further reading

RCOG Green-top guideline No. 58. *The management of vulval skin disorders*. 2011. Available at: www.gp-training.net/training/tutorials/management/audit /screen.htm

Collins S, Arulkumaran S, et al. *Oxford Handbook of Obstetrics & Gynaecology*. 3rd ed. Oxford: Oxford University Press; 2013.

30A: False – Young women usually have multifocal disease.
30B: False – Young women usually do not have any specific findings.
30C: False – VIN specifically arises in the non-hair-bearing areas.
30D: False – In certain circumstances with extensive disease skinning vulvectomy may be considered for treatment.
30E: True – Colposcopic examination of the cervix should be performed as VIN can co-exist with CIN in 20–25% of cases.

Further reading

RCOG Green-top guideline No. 58. *The management of vulval skin disorders*. 2011. Available at: www.gp-training.net/training/tutorials/management/audit/ screen.htm

Collins S, Arulkumaran S, et al. *Oxford Handbook of Obstetrics & Gynaecology*. 3rd ed. Oxford: Oxford University Press; 2013.

31A: False – HPV is a DNA virus.
31B: False – HPV is predominantly but not always transmitted by sexual contact (palmar and plantar warts).
31C: True – HPV commonly infects squamous epithelium.
31D: True – More than 100 HPV viruses have been described. High-risk HPV (type 16 and 18) are implicated in the causation of both pre-invasive lesions of the cervix and cervical cancer.
31E: True – Low-risk HPVs generally cause benign genital warts. Most common ones are HPV 6 and HPV 11.

Further reading

Collins S, Arulkumaran S, et al. *Oxford Handbook of Obstetrics & Gynaecology*. 3rd ed. Oxford: Oxford University Press; 2013.

32A: False
32B: True
32C: False
32D: False
32E: False

Further reading

Collins S, Arulkumaran S, et al. *Oxford Handbook of Obstetrics & Gynaecology.* 3rd ed. Oxford: Oxford University Press; 2013.

33A: True – BRCA2 mutation is inherited as autosomal dominant.
33B: True
33C: False – BRCA1 increases the risk of ovarian cancer by 60%.
33D: False – Endometrial cancer is not associated with BRCA1 mutation.
33E: False – HNPCC genes are associated with colorectal, endometrial and ovarian cancers.

Further reading

Collins S, Arulkumaran S, et al. *Oxford Handbook of Obstetrics & Gynaecology.* 3rd ed. Oxford: Oxford University Press; 2013.

Carpenter KM, Eisenberg S, et al. Characterizing biased cancer-related cognitive processing: relationships with BRCA1/2 genetic mutation status, personal cancer history, age, and prophylactic surgery. *Health Psychol.* 2013; [Epub ahead of print].

34A: True
34B: False – The incidence of VTE in postmenopausal women is almost double that of premenopausal women.
34C: True – The risk factors for VTE include varicose veins, malignancy, nephrotic syndrome, road traffic accidents, connective tissue diseases and HRT itself. Malignancy should be ruled out in women who are over 50 years of age and have developed VTE within the last year.
34D: False – Any women who develop VTE should be advised to stop HRT.
34E: False – Universal screening for thrombophilia is not necessary before starting HRT, unless specific risk factors for VTE are identified.

Further reading

Department of Health press release. *Further advice on safety of Hormone Replacement Therapy (HRT).* 2003. Available at: www.dh.gov.uk/en /Publicationsandstatistics/Pressreleases/DH_4062864

RCOG study group statement. *Menopause and Hormone Replacement.* 2004. Available at: www.rcog.org.uk/womens-health/clinical-guidance /menopause-and-hormone-replacement-study-group-statement

RCOG Scientific Impact Paper 6. *Alternatives to HRT for the Management of Symptoms of the Menopause.* 2010. Available at: www .rcog.org.uk/womens-health/clinical-guidance /alternatives-hrt-management-symptoms-menopause

Collins S, Arulkumaran S, et al. *Oxford Handbook of Obstetrics & Gynaecology.* 3rd ed. Oxford: Oxford University Press; 2013.

BASIC SURGICAL SKILLS – QUESTIONS

SBAs

Question 1

A 29-year-old woman presents to her GP with small lumps on her vulva. Examination reveals warty lesions. Subsequently she is referred to the vulval clinic. The biopsy of the lesions reveals benign genital warts. The following drugs can be used in the treatment of her condition except which one of the following?

A. Trichloracetic acid
B. Podophyllin
C. Podophyllotoxin
D. Dactinomycin
E. Imiquimod

Question 2

A 29-year-old woman comes to see her GP for advice as her mother, aunt and grandmother have all had ovarian cancers. Which of the following would reduce her risk of developing ovarian cancer?

A. Prophylactic bilateral salpingo-oophorectomy once family complete
B. Having knowledge about BRCA1 familial cancer
C. Monthly colour doppler ultrasound examination
D. Use of clomiphene citrate
E. Monthly measurement of Ca-125

Question 3

With regard to treatment of CIN, which one of the following statements is false?

A. Treatment of CIN 2 and 3 can be treated at first colposcopic assessment.
B. The standard treatment for CIN 2 and 3 is excisional treatment of the cervix.
C. When CIN 2 and 3 are treated at first colposcopic assessment, it should be by excisional treatment to provide specimen for histological examination.
D. CIN 1 can be treated with ablative techniques.
E. CIN 2 and 3 can be treated with cervical biopsy only.

Question 4

Which one of the following statements is true with respect to perineal tears?

A. Fourth-degree tear involves injury to the anal sphincter complex, but not anal mucosa.
B. Third-degree tear involves injury to the perineal muscle complex.
C. Intact perineal skin excludes the possibility of damage to the anal sphincter complex.
D. First-degree tear involves the skin and superficial perineal muscles.
E. The degree of trauma in a right mediolateral episiotomy is equivalent to a second-degree tear.

Question 5

A 22-year-old Caucasian para 0 woman attends maternal medicine clinic at 13 weeks' gestation following her normal dating scan. Her booking bloods are normal. She gives a history of deep venous thrombosis following a pelvic fracture after a trip over the stairs 2 years ago. Her recent thrombophilia screen is negative. Choose the most appropriate management option for this woman with regards to thrombopropylaxis.

A. TEDs only during pregnancy
B. TEDs and low molecular weight heparin (LMWH) during antenatal period
C. Aspirin during antenatal period
D. Aspirin and TED stockings during antenatal period
E. 6 weeks of postpartum LMWH

Question 6

A 39-year-old African Caribbean woman presents to her GP with menorrhagia of 10 months' duration. She does not give any history of intermenstrual or postcoital bleeding. All her previous smears have been normal. Vaginal examination reveals an essentially normal pelvis. She suffers from Crohn's disease and is taking oral sulphasalazine. She is fed up and is asking for a hysterectomy. What is her first line of management for menorrhagia?

A. Hysterectomy
B. Subtotal hysterectomy
C. Levonorgestrel-releasing intrauterine system (LNG-IUS)
D. Injectable long-acting progestogens
E. Progesterone-only pill (POP)

Question 7

A 29-year-old woman presents to the emergency department by ambulance with a history of a severe headache for 3 days and focal seizures. Two months prior to this, she presented to her GP with menorrhagia of 10 months' duration. She was offered LNG-IUS but she declined. She was prescribed tranexamic acid to be taken during her periods. Her medications box reveals that she has taken tranexamic acid for the whole previous month. There is no history of any viral illness recently. What is the likely diagnosis in her case?

A. Subarachnoid haemorrhage
B. Intracerebral haemorrhage
C. Cerebral sinus thrombosis
D. Drug-induced psychosis
E. Intracranial tumour

EMQs

OPTIONS FOR QUESTIONS 1–3

A. Uterosacral ligament
B. Transverse cervical ligament
C. Pubocervical ligament
D. Lateral cervical ligament
E. Round ligament
F. Cardinal ligament
G. Broad ligament
H. Ovarian ligament
 I. Mackenrodt's ligament
 J. Infundibulopelvic ligament

Instructions

For each clinical scenario below, choose the single most appropriate anatomical structure from the above list of options. Each option may be used once, more than once or not at all.

1. You are assisting a total abdominal hysterectomy and bilateral salpingo-oophorectomy procedure on a 58-year-old woman with complex endometrial hyperplasia. The surgeon has to clamp and cut one of the above structures to excise ovaries from the pelvic side wall.

2. A 36-year-old para 3 woman had laparoscopic sterilization one year ago. She presents with history of 6 weeks, amenorrhoea, lower abdominal pains and a positive pregnancy test. Ultrasound confirms a right-sided ectopic pregnancy and at laparoscopy, Filshie clip was found on this ligament on the right side, instead of the fallopian tube.

3. A 26-year-old nulliparous woman attends the gynaecology clinic with history of severe dysmenorrhoea and dyspareunia. On examination, the uterus is retroverted, fixed and tender with irregular nodules in the pouch of Douglas. Ultrasound shows right endometrioma measuring 5 × 5 cm. At laparoscopy, you notice extensive endometriosis on these structures obliterating the pouch of Douglas.

OPTIONS FOR QUESTIONS 4–6

A. Capacity
B. Beneficence
C. Competence
D. Assault
E. Battery
F. Negligence
G. Gillick competent or meeting the Fraser guidelines
H. Bolam test
I. Confidentiality
J. Autonomy

Instructions

For each clinical scenario below, choose the single most appropriate principle from the above list of options. Each option may be used once, more than once or not at all.

4. A 36-year-old para 5 woman is a practicing Jehovah's witness and has signed the advanced directive declining blood transfusion under any circumstances. She had five normal deliveries in the past and had uncomplicated antenatal period during this pregnancy. She had a precipitate labour with massive postpartum haemorrhage (PPH). Despite prompt resuscitation and appropriate management of the PPH, she dies.

5. A 38-year-old woman with a previous caesarean section presents in active labour at term and wishes to have vaginal birth after caesarean section. At 8 cm dilatation, there is fetal bradycardia followed by maternal hypovolemia and loss of consciousness. After making the decision that this patient is not in a fit state to consent, you proceed with an emergency laparotomy.

6. After an episode of unprotected intercourse a 15-year-old girl attends the family planning clinic for emergency contraception. As she has been sexually active for the last 3 months she is also requesting a reliable contraceptive method. Her family is unaware of her relationship and she does not want to disclose.

OPTIONS FOR QUESTIONS 7–9

A. Atelectasis
B. Pulmonary embolism
C. Paralytic ileus
D. Bowel perforation
E. Uterine dehiscence
F. Endometritis
G. Infected pelvic collection
H. Uterine perforation
I. Small bowel obstruction
J. Ureteric injury

Instructions

For each clinical scenario below, choose the single most likely surgical complication from the above list of options. Each may be used once, more than once or not at all.

7. A 26-year-old woman attends the emergency department with a history of lower abdominal pain and feeling unwell, 5 days after an emergency caesarean section for failure to progress in the second stage after a failed instrumental delivery. Estimated blood loss at delivery was 1500 ml. She recovered well postoperatively and was discharged on day 3. Her pulse was 112, BP 100/60 mmHg, temperature 38.6°C, respiratory rate 20 and oxygen saturation 98%. On examination, she was tender in the lower abdomen with guarding and bowel sounds were present. Her WBC was 16 and CRP 250. Though there is some clinical improvement after admission with intravenous antibiotics, she still has swinging temperatures.

8. A 34-year-old woman with a BMI of 40 attends the emergency department with a history of sudden onset of left abdominal pain and fever with rigors, ten days postoperatively after an emergency caesarean section for failure to progress in the second stage after failed instrumental delivery. At delivery, there was an extension of the left uterine angle with massive haemorrhage, which was controlled by placing multiple haemostatic sutures and securing uterine angles. Her pulse is 116, BP 110/80 mmHg and temperature 38°C. On examination, there is tenderness in the left lower abdomen and left flank. Her WBC is 15 and CRP is 110.

9. A 28-year-old woman attends the emergency department with severe lower abdominal pain and feeling unwell, on day 2 after a diagnostic laparoscopy for chronic pelvic pain and subfertility. Her pulse is 114, BP 110/70 mmHg and temperature is 37°C. On examination, there is severe tenderness in the lower abdomen with rigidity, guarding and rebound tenderness. Her WBC is 19 and CRP is 170.

MCQs

1. A 20-year-old woman attends the gynaecology clinic with pelvic pain. After assessment she is booked for diagnostic laparoscopy. She is nulliparous and her BMI is 20. The following blood vessels may be injured at diagnostic laparoscopy:
   A. Abdominal aorta
   B. Internal mammary artery
   C. Inferior epigastic artery
   D. Right phrenic artery
   E. Inferior mesenteric artery

2. The risk factors for utero-vaginal prolapse include:
   A. Nulliparity
   B. Childbirth
   C. Obesity
   D. Chronic constipation
   E. Pelvic inflammatory disease

3. Women with genitourinary prolapse may present with:
   A. Recurrent UTIs
   B. Haematuria
   C. Dragging sensation on standing
   D. Pain during intercourse
   E. Recurrent miscarriage

4. The following treatments have been used in the management of utero-vaginal prolapse:
   A. Abdominal belt
   B. Vaginal shelf pessaries
   C. Vaginal cones to increase pelvic floor muscle strength
   D. Surgery to correct prolapse
   E. Duloxetene to increase pelvic floor muscle strength

5. The uses of botulinum toxin in medicine include:
   A. Overactive bladder
   B. To prevent development of wrinkles
   C. To prevent muscle spasms following breast reconstruction
   D. Treatment of gastritis
   E. Treatment of ectopic pregnancy

6. The following are standard treatment modalities used to treat stage 1a grade 1 endometrioid adenocarcinoma of the uterus:
   A. Laparotomy, total abdominal hysterectomy and bilateral salpingo-oophorectomy
   B. Laparoscopic assisted vaginal hysterectomy and bilateral salpingo-oophorectomy
   C. High dose progestogens
   D. Primary pelvic radiotherapy
   E. Chemotherapy

7. Bowel injury in gynaecological surgery:
   A. Is more common with abdominal hysterectomy than vaginal hysterectomy
   B. Is a very common complication
   C. Incidence is as high as 10%
   D. Is more common with laparoscopic hysterectomy than abdominal hysterectomy
   E. May go unnoticed at the time of surgery

8. The following treatments are described for the treatment of vulval intraepithelial neoplasia (VIN):
   A. Partial vulvectomy
   B. Local excision
   C. Skinning vulvectomy
   D. Laser vapourization
   E. Radical vulvectomy

9. A 29-year-old para 1 woman presents to the emergency department with a history of 6 weeks' amenorrhoea and abdominal pain. Her pregnancy test is positive. Her observations are stable. She is admitted to the gynaecology ward. She has a transvaginal scan the following day that reveals a 3 cm ectopic pregnancy in the left fallopian tube. The following treatments can be offered to this woman:
   A. Laparoscopic unilateral salpingectomy
   B. Laparoscopic unilateral salpingostomy
   C. Midline laparotomy and unilateral salpingectomy
   D. Laparoscopic bilateral salpingectomy
   E. Laparotomy and bilateral salpingectomy

10. The following women need caesarean section for delivery of their baby:
    A. A 29-year-old para 2 woman (previous 2 normal deliveries) presents to the labour ward at 36 weeks' gestation with SROM.
    B. A 38-year-old para 1 woman presents to labour ward at 34 weeks' gestation with regular painful contractions. Her ultrasound scan at 20 weeks' gestation shows placenta covering the cervical os completely.
    C. A 28-year-old para 1 woman attends the antenatal clinic at 34 weeks' gestation. She is requesting caesarean section as she had forceps delivery during her last pregnancy.
    D. A 29-year-old para 1 woman presents to the labour ward at 39 weeks' gestation with regular painful contractions. Vaginal examination reveals 3 cm cervical dilatation. While performing vaginal examination you notice multiple vesicular lesions on bilateral labia and mons pubis consistent with primary active genital herpes infection.
    E. A 38-year-old para 1 woman presents to the labour ward at 38 weeks' gestation with painful labour contractions. She is on anti-retroviral drug therapy and her recent viral load is >500 RNA copies.

11. With regard to treatment of fibroids:
    A. Transcervical resection of fibroids (TCRF) is associated with increased morbidity compared to open myomectomy.
    B. Open myomectomy is associated with an increased operative morbidity compared to open hysterectomy.
    C. Uterine artery embolization (UAE) is not recommended in nulliparous women as it is associated with decline in ovarian function.
    D. Transcervical resection of fibroids is sometimes associated with fluid overload.
    E. The use of GnRH analogues before myomectomy not only reduces the size of the fibroids but also reduces blood loss and operating surgical time.

12. The following are the correct classifications for the urgency of caesarean section in these clinical scenarios:
    A. A 29-year-old para 1 woman presents to the labour ward at 39 weeks' gestation with a history of spontaneous rupture of membranes (SROM). Midwife performs speculum examination, which reveals 3 cm cervical dilatation and umbilical cord in the vagina. Fetal heartbeat is 100 bpm by auscultation method. This should be performed as a category 1 caesarean section.
    B. A 29-year-old para 1 woman presents to labour ward at 39 weeks' gestation with a history of antepartum haemorrhage (APH). Abdominal examination reveals a tense and tender uterus and speculum examination reveals active vaginal bleeding. Fetal heart beat is 110 per minute. Her ultrasound scan at 20 weeks shows fundal placenta. This should be performed as category 3 caesarean section.
    C. A 29-year-old para 1 woman (previous 1 LSCS) presents to the labour ward at 39 weeks' gestation with SROM. Otherwise she is clinically stable. She is booked for elective caesarean section in 3 days' time. This should be performed as a category 1 caesarean section.
    D. A 29-year-old nulliparous woman at 37 weeks' gestation had a failed external cephalic version (ECV) for breech presentation. She is keen to have caesarean section and this should be performed as a category 2 caesarean section.
    E. A 29-year-old para 1 woman presents to the labour ward at 39 weeks' gestation with history of SROM. Abdominal examination reveals regular contractions. Speculum examination confirms 1 cm cervical dilatation, SROM and thin meconium stained liquor. Therefore, she is commenced on a CTG for fetal monitoring, which is normal. Twenty-four hours later vaginal examination reveals no progress in cervical dilatation. A decision to perform caesarean section is made. This should be performed as a category 3 caesarean section.

13. The following should be discussed when counselling a woman with one previous uncomplicated caesarean section wanting to try for a vaginal birth:
    A. Chances of successful planned vaginal birth after caesarean section (VBAC) are 90–95%.
    B. VBAC carries a risk of uterine rupture of 1 in 200.
    C. Women should be informed that there is virtually no risk of uterine rupture in women undergoing elective caesarean section.
    D. Planned VBAC compared with elective repeat caesarean section (ERCS) carries around 1% additional risk of blood transfusion or endometritis.
    E. VBAC carries an 8/100 risk of the infant developing hypoxic ischaemic encephalopathy.

14. The following signs may indicate scar dehiscence in women with previous caesarean section:
    A. Maternal tachycardia
    B. Normal CTG
    C. Presence of uterine contractions
    D. Sudden loss of fetal heart
    E. Vaginal bleeding

15. A 29-year-old para 1 woman presents to the early pregnancy assessment unit (EPAU) at 8 weeks' gestation with mild vaginal bleeding. A transvaginal ultrasound scan performed by ultrasonographer reveals an absent fetal heart beat and is reported as missed miscarriage. You are on gynaecology on call and you have been asked to review this woman and consent her for surgical evacuation of retained products of conception (ERPC). The following risks should be discussed with this woman:
    A. One in 1000 women require a repeat surgical evacuation.
    B. Three in 1000 women will have a localized pelvic infection.
    C. Three in 10 women would need blood transfusion.
    D. Bleeding following ERPC may last up to 2 weeks.
    E. Uterine perforation is uncommon but may be seen in 5 in 1000 women.

4

BASIC SURGICAL SKILLS – ANSWERS

SBAs

Answer 1: D

- Genital warts are usually a clinical diagnosis. They can cause discomfort and psychological trauma.
- Women with genital warts should be referred to genitourinary clinics for treatment and also should be screened for other sexually transmitted genital infections.
- Most warts resolve spontaneously.

Treatment of Genital Warts

Medical Treatment	
Podophyllin	Used for local application on vulva and perianal region
Podophyllotoxin	Used for local application on vulva and perianal region
Imiquimod	Immune modifying agent
Interferons	Immune modifying agent
Trichloracetic acid (TCA)	Used for local application on vagina and cervical warts
Fluorouracil (5-FU)	Used locally
Caution: podophyllin, podophyllotoxin and 5-flurouracil are contraindicated during pregnancy. Trichloracetic acid and imiquimod can be safely used during pregnancy.	
Surgical Treatment	
Surgical excision	Can be used for small as well as large warts
	Can be used for warts resistant to drug
	Safe in pregnancy
Cryotherapy	Can be used in pregnancy
Laser treatment (vaporization)	More expensive

Further reading

Lazaro N. *Sexually Transmitted Infections in Primary Care*. 2nd ed. RCGP/BASHH. 2013. Available at: www.bashh.org/documents/Sexually%20Transmitted%20 Infections%20in%20Primary%20Care%202013.pdf

Answer 2: A

Women should be appropriately counselled about the risk:benefit ratio of prophylactic bilateral salpingo-oophorectomy. On one hand this results in premature menopause and on the other hand it reduces the risk of ovarian cancer by 95%. Women should be informed that there is still a 2% (1 in 50) risk of primary peritoneal cancer, which behaves similar to ovarian cancer. The risk of ovarian cancer in women with BRCA1 and BRCA2 is 50–60% (1 in 2) and 30% (1 in 3) respectively. This risk actually starts around the age of 40 in women with BRCA1 and in the mid-40s in women with BRCA2 carriers; therefore, these women should be advised to complete their families earlier and bilateral salpingo-oophorectomy advised in the future at the above ages.

These women should also be counselled about early menopause and HRT options available to them. If HRT is started following oophorectomy, it should be stopped around the age of 51 as the risk of breast cancer is increased with HRT.

If women are BRCA1 or BRCA2 carriers and are using the combined oral contraceptive pill (COCP) for contraception, they should be advised to use alternatives (progestogen-only contraception e.g. Mirena, Implanon, POPs and copper IUD) as COCP slightly increases the risk of breast cancer. At the same time they should be informed that their risk of developing ovarian cancer is reduced by 50% if they had used COCP previously.

Prophylactic bilateral salpingo-oophorectomy should be considered in women:

- around the age of 40 years in women with BRCA1 carrier;
- around the age of 45 years in women with BRCA2 carrier;
- if there is strong family history of cancer as above but unable to perform gene testing; or
- if they are positive for BRCA1 and BRCA2 gene (if screen positive may consider prophylactic mastectomy and also other family members should be counselled and genetically screened for BRCA1 and BRCA2 gene).

Further reading

Moorman PG, Havrilesky LJ, et al. Oral contraceptives and risk of ovarian cancer and breast cancer among high-Risk women: A systematic review and meta-analysis. *J Clin Oncol.* 2013 Oct 21. [Epub ahead of print].

Gadducci A, Sergiampietri C, Tana R. Alternatives to risk-reducing surgery for ovarian cancer. *Ann Oncol.* 2013 Nov; 24 Suppl 8:viii47–viii53.

Finch A, Bacopulos S, et al. Preventing ovarian cancer through genetic testing: a population-based study. *Clin Genet.* 2013 Nov 6; doi: 10.1111/cge.12313. [Epub ahead of print].

Answer 3: E

Treatment and treatment methods of CIN

- CIN 1: ablative or excisional [Large loop excision of transformation zone (LLETZ)] methods. This can be performed under local anaesthetic in the clinic or under general anaesthetic in special circumstances (e.g. anxious patient, large lesion, large transformation zone, patient not willing to have the procedure under local anaesthetic).
- CIN 2 and 3: usually excisional methods (LLETZ, knife or laser cone). When the treatment occurs at first visit in colposcopy, it is known as 'see and treat', otherwise the treatment is performed at a later visit when the biopsy results are available.
- LLETZ can be performed under local or general anaesthetic. Laser cone can be performed under local anaesthetic but knife cone biopsy is usually performed under general anaesthesia. Cone biopsy is also a treatment for cervical glandular intraepithelial neoplasia (CGIN).
- Hysterectomy is performed when CIN is associated with other gynaecological conditions or if the excision treatment of CIN fails.

Ablative methods of treatment

- Laser vaporization of the tissue: performed under local anaesthetic.
- Cryotherapy is freezing the tissue: performed under local anaesthetic.
- Cold coagulation involves boiling of tissue by heated probe (100–120°C): performed under local anaesthetic.
- Radical electrodiathermy involves burning of the transformation zone: performed under general anaesthesia.

Further reading

NHSCSP Publication No. 20. *Colposcopy and Programme Management. Guidelines for the NHS Cervical Screening Programme.* 2nd ed. 2010. Available at: www.bsccp.org.uk/colposcopy-resources /colposcopy-and-programme-management-1

Answer 4: E

Perineal tears classification: first degree, injury to perineal skin only; second degree, injury to perineal muscles; third degree, injury to the anal sphincter complex; and fourth degree, anal sphincter complex and anal epithelium.

Further reading

RCOG Green-top guideline No. 29. *Management of third- and fourth-degree perineal tears.* 2001. Available at: www.rcog.org.uk/womens-health/clinical-guidance /management-third-and-fourth-degree-perineal-tears-green-top-29

Answer 5: E

Management of pregnant women with past history of VTE

- All women should be assessed at their booking visit for risk factors for VTE. This should be revisited at every interaction during the antenatal period, emergency admission, before or during labour. All women should be encouraged to mobilize during labour and the puerperium. Dehydration should be avoided.

- In women with a history of a previous single episode of VTE (not oestrogen related e.g. road traffic accident) and in the absence of other risk factors, it may be reasonable to offer antenatal surveillance (antenatal LMWH is not routinely recommended). However, these women should be offered postpartum thromboprophylaxis with LMWH.

- Women with a history of recurrent previous VTE should be offered thromboprophylaxis with LMWH antenatally and for at least 6 weeks postpartum.

- Women with a history of previous VTE and a family history of VTE in a first-degree relative should be offered thromboprophylaxis with LMWH antenatally and for at least 6 weeks postpartum.

- Women with previous recurrent VTE or a previous unprovoked or oestrogen- or pregnancy-related VTE should be offered thromboprophylaxis with LMWH antenatally and for at least 6 weeks postpartum.

- Women with previous VTE and documented thrombophilia should be offered thromboprophylaxis with LMWH antenatally and for at least 6 weeks postpartum.

- Women with three or more persisting risk factors should be considered for thromboprophylaxis with LMWH antenatally and for at least 6 weeks postpartum.

- Women with two or more persistent risk factors should be considered for LMWH for 7 days following delivery. (Age over 35 years and BMI greater than 30/body weight greater than 90 kg are independent risk factors for postpartum VTE even if the woman had vaginal delivery.) The combination of either of these risk factors with any other risk factor for VTE (such as pre-eclampsia or immobility) or the presence of two other persisting risk factors is an indication for use of LMWH for 7 days postpartum.

Further reading

RCOG Green-top guideline No. 37a. *Thrombosis and embolism during pregnancy and the puerperium, reducing the risk.* 2009. Available at: www.rcog.org.uk /womens-health/clinical-guidance/reducing-risk-of-thrombosis-greentop37a

Answer 6: C

Menorrhagia is defined as regular heavy periods for six consecutive cycles with no IMB or PCB and has a normal cervical smear.

Heavy menstrual bleeding (HMB) can be defined as excessive menstrual blood loss that interferes with a woman's physical, social, emotional and/or material quality of life (NICE).

Treatment should be considered in the following order:

- Levonorgestrel-releasing intrauterine system (LNG-IUS) is first-line treatment
- Tranexamic acid or non-steroidal anti-inflammatory drugs (NSAIDs)
- Combined oral contraceptives (COCs) depending on age
- Norethisterone (15 mg) daily from days 5 to 26
- Injected long-acting progestogens

Further reading

NICE clinical guideline No. 44. *Heavy menstrual bleeding.* 2007. Available at: www .nice.org.uk/nicemedia/pdf/CG44NICEGuideline.pdf

Answer 7: C

Tranexamic acid is a synthetic derivative of the amino acid lysine. It has traditionally been used to treat or prevent excessive blood loss during surgery. In gynaecology it is used in the treatment of menorrhagia. It is an antifibrinolytic agent that competitively inhibits the activation of plasminogen to plasmin, thus preventing fibrinolysis.

The side effects are less common but are mainly gastrointestinal. These include dizziness, fatigue, headache and hypersensitivity reactions. The use of tranexamic acid also has a potential risk of thrombosis. The US Food and Drug Administration (FDA) has approved tranexamic acid in the form of oral tablets for the treatment of heavy menstrual bleeding.

The clinical presentation of women with cerebral venous thrombosis can be varied. The most frequent presentation is headache and focal seizures. In this case, the likely diagnosis is cerebral venous thrombosis as tranexamic acid is a risk factor. The doctor who prescribes this medication should clearly explain to the woman that the drug should be taken during menstrual periods and not indefinitely.

The other drugs that are implicated in cerebral venous thrombosis are COCP, HRT, androgens, ecstasy and L-asparaginase.

Further reading

NICE clinical guideline No. 44. *Heavy menstrual bleeding.* 2007. Available at: www.nice.org.uk/nicemedia/pdf/CG44NICEGuideline.pdf

EMQs

Answers 1–3

1. J

Infundibulopelvic ligament, also known as suspensory ligament of the ovary, is a fold of peritoneum extending out from the ovary to the pelvic side wall.

2. E

This structure, very close and anterior to the fallopian tube, is the round ligament. One should be cautious in ensuring that the fallopian tube is clipped, not the round ligament, by identifying the fimbrial end and following the tube to the uterine cornua.

3. A

Endometriosis commonly affects the uterosacral ligaments and the nodules are often palpable on vaginal examination, through the posterior fornix.

Further reading

Collins S, Arulkumaran S, et al. *Oxford Handbook of Obstetrics & Gynaecology.* 3rd ed. Oxford: Oxford University Press; 2013.

Answers 4–6

4. J

Autonomy: the patient has the right to accept or refuse medical treatment, even if the consequences are detrimental to their health, as long as they are competent and able to make informed decisions.

5. B

Beneficence is action taken in the best interests of the patient to prevent significant harm or death when informed consent is not obtainable. In this clinical scenario, uterine rupture is the likely diagnosis and laparotomy is performed in the patient's best interest in order to prevent the maternal and fetal demise, even though consent was not obtained.

6. G

Gillick competence or Fraser guidelines: children under the age of 16 may have the capacity to consent to treatment, though they cannot refuse treatment.

Further reading

Wheeler, R. Gillick or Fraser? A plea for consistency over competence in children: Gillick and Fraser are not interchangeable. *BMJ.* 2006; 332(7545):807.

DeCruz SP. Parents, doctors and children: the Gillick case and beyond. *J Social Welfare Law.* 1987;93–108.

Collins S, Arulkumaran S, et al. *Oxford Handbook of Obstetrics & Gynaecology.* 3rd ed. Oxford: Oxford University Press; 2013.

Answers 7–9

7. G
Infected pelvic collection is the likely diagnosis in this case, in view of the difficult second-stage caesarean section with postpartum haemorrhage and the fact that all of the symptoms and signs are localized to the lower abdomen. The pelvic hematoma gets infected and, if proven, needs to be drained either surgically or under radiological guidance.

8. J
The likely diagnosis in this clinical scenario is ureteric injury, given the clinical picture and surgical details of extension of uterine angle and multiple haemostatic sutures near the uterine angles, where the ureters are in close proximity to the uterine arteries.

9. D
Bowel perforation is the likely diagnosis and should be ruled out in this clinical scenario, where the woman is unwell with acute abdomen post laparoscopy.

Further reading

Collins S, Arulkumaran S, et al. *Oxford Handbook of Obstetrics & Gynaecology.* 3rd ed. Oxford: Oxford University Press; 2013.

MCQs

1A: True
1B: False
1C: True
1D: False
1E: False

Further reading

RCOG Green-top guideline No. 49. *Laparoscopic injuries*. 2008.
    Available at www.rcog.org.uk/womens-health/clinical-guidance
    /preventing-entry-related-gynaecological-laparoscopic-injuries-green-top-49

2A: False
2B: True
2C: True
2D: True
2E: False

Risk factors for utero-vaginal prolapse include:

- Conditions giving rise to the increased intra-abdominal pressure: obesity, constipation and chronic cough
- Structural weakness of the pelvic floor: childbirth, menopause

Further reading

Collins S, Arulkumaran S, et al. *Oxford Handbook of Obstetrics & Gynaecology*.
    3rd ed. Oxford: Oxford University Press; 2013.

3A: True
3B: False
3C: True
3D: True
3E: False

The following may be elicited in women with a history of genitourinary prolapse:

- Stress incontinence/pelvic floor disruption
- Dragging sensation on standing
- Something coming out of vagina or 'like my insides are falling out'
- Pain during intercourse/dyspareunia
- Symptom exacerbated by gravity
- Recurrent UTIs secondary to incomplete emptying
- Difficulty in defaecation
- Urinary retention and overflow incontinence due to prolapse
- Injuries to the back and neurological problems

Further reading

Collins S, Arulkumaran S, et al. *Oxford Handbook of Obstetrics & Gynaecology*. 3rd ed. Oxford: Oxford University Press; 2013.

4A: False
4B: True
4C: True
4D: True
4E: False – Duloxetene is used for the treatment of stress incontinence. It is second-line therapy for treating stress incontinence if surgery for any reason cannot be performed. Suicidal tendency is known to increase in women who use Duloxetene.

Further reading

www.patient.co.uk Health Information. *Genitourinary prolapse*. Available at: www .patient.co.uk/health/Genitourinary-GU-Prolapse.htm

NICE Guidelines. *Surgical repair of vaginal wall prolapse using mesh*. 2008. Available at: publications.nice.org.uk/surgical-repair-of-vaginal-wall -prolapse-using-mesh-ipg267

Collins S, Arulkumaran S, et al. *Oxford Handbook of Obstetrics & Gynaecology*. 3rd ed. Oxford: Oxford University Press; 2013.

5A: True
5B: True
5C: True
5D: False
5E: False

Botulinum toxin is a protein and neurotoxin produced by the bacterium *clostridium botulinum*. It acts by decreasing the muscle activity by blocking the release of acetylcholine from the neurone. This will weaken the muscle effectively for a period of 4–6 months.

The toxin can be injected into the head and neck to treat chronic headaches and migraine. In women with an overactive bladder, after all the treatments are exhausted, botulinum toxin can be used for treatment. However, it may have to be repeated every 6 months as its action wears off. Some women may go into retention of urine and may need long-term self intermittent catheterization. Therefore, women have to be counselled appropriately before considering this option for treatment.

The other uses of botulinum toxin include:

- Cerebral palsy
- Cervical dystonia
- Anal fissure
- Hyperhidrosis or excessive sweating
- Strabismus
- Bhlepharospasm

- Achalasia
- Vaginismus
- Neurogenic bladder
- Vocal cord dysfunction
- Parkinson disease
- Multiple sclerosis

Further reading

Collins S, Arulkumaran S, et al. *Oxford Handbook of Obstetrics & Gynaecology*. 3rd ed. Oxford: Oxford University Press; 2013.

6A: True – The standard treatment for endometrial tumours is hysterectomy and bilateral salpingo-oophorectomy (BSO) and peritoneal washings.
6B: True – Hysterectomy and BSO can be performed by lapartotomy or laparoscopically.
6C: False – High dose progestogens is a short term option in young women who wish to preserve fertility but not standard treatment used for treating endometrial cancer.
6D: True – Radiotherapy as a primary modality of treatment is not a standard treatment. Around 80% of endometrial cancers are diagnosed early and amenable to surgical treatment.
6E: False – Chemotherapy is generally not used for such low-grade tumours.

Further reading

Collins S, Arulkumaran S, et al. *Oxford Handbook of Obstetrics & Gynaecology*. 3rd ed. Oxford: Oxford University Press; 2013.

7A: True – Abdominal surgery is associated with increased risk of bowel damage than vaginal surgery.
7B: False
7C: False – The incidence of damage is 0.3–0.8%.
7D: False – Abdominal surgery is associated with increased risk of bowel damage than laparoscopic surgery.
7E: True – If the bowel injury is noticed at the time of surgery it can be repaired immediately. If it goes unnoticed at the time of surgery, which is usually the case, the patient manifests symptoms on day 2–3 of the postoperative period. Depending on the extent and site of bowel damage, patients may present with abdominal pain or distension, vomiting, swinging pyrexia, signs of peritonism (abdominal guarding, rigidity, tenderness and rebound tenderness) with or without signs of septic shock. Abdominal X-ray may show gas under the diaphragm or distended loops of bowel. CT scan with contrast may further help to localize the bowel damage and collection due to leak.

Further reading

Amer SA. Postoperative care. Shaw RW, Luesley D, Monga A (eds). *Gynaecology*. 4th ed. Edinburgh: Churchill Livingstone; 2010. Chapter 9.

8A: True
8B: True
8C: True
8D: True
8E: False

Types of VIN, Risk Factors and Treatment of VIN

Differentiated Type VIN	Classic or Usual Type VIN
More common in the age group 60–80 years	More common in women in their 30s and 40s
Not related to HPV infection	HPV related
Commonly associated with lichen sclerosus and may be associated with lichen planus	Associated with Bowen's disease
Both VIN and lichen sclerosus or lichen planus are seen next to each other	Classified into warty, basaloid and mixed pathological subtypes
Usually unifocal disease	Usually multifocal disease, can be associated with CIN and VAIN
Malignant potential is high	Other risk factors include smoking, sexual promiscuity and immunosuppression
Therapies such as antiviral and vaccination are unlikely to be successful treatment or preventive strategies	Topical imiquimod, an immune-response modifier, is an effective method for treatment of genital warts and has been used for VIN. Surgical treatment methods for VIN include local excision, partial vulvectomy and skinning vulvectomy.

VIN is associated with other lower genital tract intraepithelial neoplasia including cervical intraepithelial neoplasia (CIN), vaginal intraepithelial neoplasia (VAIN) and anal intraepithelial neoplasia (AIN).

Further reading

RCOG Green-top guideline No. 58. *Vulval skin disorders, Management.* 2011. Available at: www.rcog.org.uk/womens-health/clinical-guidance /management-vulval-skin-disorders-green-top-58

Collins S, Arulkumaran S, et al. *Oxford Handbook of Obstetrics & Gynaecology.* 3rd ed. Oxford: Oxford University Press; 2013.

9A: True
9B: True
9C: False
9D: False
9E: False

The conventional treatment for ectopic pregnancy was laparotomy and salpingectomy. This stands true in the current practice only if the woman is haemodynamically unstable and the person who is operating does not have appropriate training in laparoscopy.

Currently, a laparoscopic approach is used for treating ectopic pregnancy in the fallopian tube. RCOG recommends laparoscopic salpingectomy if the contralateral fallopian tube is normal and laparoscopic salpingostomy if the contralateral fallopian tube is abnormal.

Further reading

RCOG Green-top guideline No. 21. *Management of tubal pregnancy.* 2004. Available at: www.rcog.org.uk/womens-health/clinical-guidance /management-tubal-pregnancy-21-may-2004

Collins S, Arulkumaran S, et al. *Oxford Handbook of Obstetrics & Gynaecology.* 3rd ed. Oxford: Oxford University Press; 2013.

10A: False – Women with previous normal deliveries can be allowed to have a vaginal delivery following SROM provided the position of the fetus is cephalic. The presence of breech presentation would require appropriate counselling with regards to mode of delivery (vaginal or caesarean section).

10B: True – Central or major placenta praevia (grade 4) is an absolute indication for caesarean section. Placenta praevia is graded as follows:

Grade 1: the distal edge of the placenta is within 2 cm of the internal os (does not reach the internal os).
Grade 2: placenta reaches the internal but does not cover it.
Grade 3: placenta covers the internal os partially.
Grade 4: placenta covers the internal os completely.

The incidence of low-lying placenta is around 20% at 20 weeks. As the uterus grows, the lower segment forms and the placenta appears to migrate upwards as the lower segment has developed below it. The incidence therefore falls to around 1–2% at 34–36 weeks. Therefore, it is important to repeat ultrasound at 34–36 weeks of gestation for placental localization. If the placenta has migrated up, then the woman can be allowed vaginal delivery. If the placenta is still low at this stage, then she would need caesarean section at 38–39 weeks' depending on the grade of placenta praevia. If these women present with heavy vaginal bleeding before the planned date of delivery, emergency caesarean section should be performed and this has to be under senior or consultant supervision.

10C: False – Previous forceps delivery is not an indication for caesarean section during the current pregnancy. One should discourage this method of delivery if there is no valid clinical reason. Careful discussion of the benefits and risks of both methods will allow making an informed choice. Written information in the form of leaflets should also be provided for the woman.

10D: True – RCOG recommends caesarean section in the presence of primary active genital herpes in order to reduce neonatal transmission.

10E: True – Anti-retroviral therapy along with caesarean section can reduce the vertical transmission rate of HIV to less than 1% in the neonate. The risk of fetal transmission is negligible when the viral load is zero or less than 50 RNA copies. In such women, vaginal delivery can be allowed. If the viral load is high as seen in the current case, caesarean section is indicated.

Further reading

RCOG Green-top guideline No. 27. *Placenta praevia, placenta praevia accreta and vasa praevia: Diagnosis and management.* 2011. Available at: www .rcog.org.uk/womens-health/clinical-guidance /placenta-praevia-and-placenta-praevia-accreta-diagnosis-and-manageme

RCOG Green-top guideline No. 39. *HIV in pregnancy, management.* 2010. Available at: www.rcog.org.uk/womens-health/clinical-guidance /management-hiv-pregnancy-green-top-39

RCOG Green-top guideline No. 30. *Genital herpes in pregnancy, management.* 2007. Available at: www.rcog.org.uk/womens-health/clinical-guidance /management-genital-herpes-pregnancy-green-top-30

11A: False – TCRF is a vaginal surgery and most patients can go home on the same day. It is associated with less morbidity than open myomectomy.
11B: False – It is debatable as long-term morbidity may be different for both operations, although both are performed by laparotomy.
11C: True – There are reports of premature ovarian failure in women who have had UAE in the reproductive age group. Therefore, this method is not recommended for use in young women, especially if they want to preserve fertility.
11D: True – Fluid media is used to distend the cavity of the uterus during the operation. This can be absorbed via open uterine veins and can lead to fluid overload. Therefore, one has to be careful and regularly assess fluid input and output during the procedure. If the negative balance is >1000 mL, the recommendation is to stop the procedure as this can be associated with electrolyte imbalance (hyponatremia). Such women would need a blood test to measure electrolytes and overnight observation in the hospital.
11E: False – The use of GnRH analogues prior to myomectomy has not been shown to reduce blood loss or operating time.

Further reading

RCOG other guidelines and reports. *Uterine Artery Embolisation in the Management of Fibroids.* 3rd ed. 2013. Available at: www.rcog.org.uk/womens-health /clinical-guidance/uterine-artery-embolisation-management-fibroids

12A: True
12B: False – This should be performed as a category 1 caesarean section, as the likely diagnosis is APH secondary to abruption.
12C: False – This should be performed as a category 3 caesarean section.
12D: False – This should be performed as a category 4 caesarean section.
12E: False – This should be performed as a category 2 caesarean section.

Classification for urgency of caesarean section

- Category 1 (Crash) emergency caesarean section: caesarean section should be performed immediately as there is immediate threat to maternal or fetal life (decision to delivery interval should be less than 30 minutes) e.g. massive antepartum haemorrhage, placental abruption, prolonged fetal bradycardia, cord prolapse, fetal compromise (fetal blood sampling pH <7.20) and uterine rupture.
- Category 2 (Urgent) emergency caesarean section: maternal or fetal compromise that is not immediately life threatening (decision to delivery interval within 60 minutes) e.g. failure to progress.
- Category 3 (Semi-elective): requires early delivery but no immediate maternal or fetal compromise (decision to delivery interval can vary depending on fetal and labour ward condition) e.g. previous LSCS with SROM (can wait until the labour ward is less busy or even till the next day if she does not go into labour and intrauterine fetal growth restriction).
- Category 4 (Elective) emergency caesarean section: performed at a suitable time to suit both the woman and the maternity services e.g. planned caesarean sections for previous caesarean sections, breech presentations, placenta praevia.

Further reading

RCOG Good Practice No. 11. *Classification of urgency of caesarean section – a continuum of risk*. 2010. Available at: www.rcog.org.uk /classification-of-urgency-of-caesarean-section-good-practice-11

13A: False – Chances of successful planned VBAC are 72–76%. Also, VBAC probably reduces the risk that their baby will have respiratory problems after birth: rates are 2–3% with planned VBAC and 3–4% with elective caesarean section. Epidural is not contraindicated with VBAC and continuous electronic fetal monitoring should be commenced following the onset of uterine contractions for the duration of planned VBAC.
13B: True – 1 in 200 or <1% or 2–7/1000 or 22–74/10,000
13C: True
13D: True
13E: False – VBAC carries an 8/10,000 risk of the infant developing hypoxic ischaemic encephalopathy. Women considering planned VBAC should be informed that there is additional risk of birth-related perinatal death (2–3/10,000) when compared with ERCS. The absolute risk of such birth-related perinatal loss is comparable to the risk for women having their first birth.

Further reading

RCOG Green-top guideline No. 45. *Birth after previous caesarean birth*. 2007. Available at: www.rcog.org.uk/womens-health/clinical-guidance /birth-after-previous-caesarean-birth-green-top-45

14A: True
14B: False
14C: False
14D: True
14E: True

The other signs that may indicate scar dehiscence include:

- suprapubic pain despite effective epidural analgesia;
- tenderness in suprapubic region;
- severe abdominal pain;
- maternal shock and collapse;
- haematuria;
- cessation of uterine contractions; and
- abnormal CTG.

Further reading

RCOG Green-top guideline No. 45. *Birth after previous caesarean birth*. 2007. Available at: www.rcog.org.uk/womens-health/clinical-guidance /birth-after-previous-caesarean-birth-green-top-45

ACOG Practice bulletin. Vaginal birth after caesarean section. Clinical management guidelines. *Int J Gynaecol Obstet*. 1999; 66: 197–204.

15A: False
15B: False
15C: False
15D: True
15E: True

Risks associated with surgical ERPC

- Frequent risks
  - Bleeding that lasts for up to 2 weeks is very common
  - 1–2 in 1000 women need blood transfusion (uncommon)
  - Five in 100 women need repeat surgical evacuation (common)
  - Three in 100 women may get localized pelvic infection (common)
- Serious risks
  - The risk of uterine perforation is up to five in 1000 women (uncommon)
  - Severe trauma to the cervix (rare)
- There is no evidence that this procedure would affect future fertility in these women

This woman should be informed about the available alternative treatments, which include medical management (with mifepristone, prostaglandins) and expectant management, particularly for women without an intact sac. They should be informed that there is still 15–50% possibility of eventually needing surgical evacuation for clinical needs or because the woman prefers to have it.

Further reading

RCOG consent advice No. 10. *Surgical evacuation of the uterus for early pregnancy loss.* 2010. Available at: www.rcog.org.uk /surgical-evacuation-uterus-early-pregnancy-loss-consent-advice-10

5

ANTENATAL CARE – QUESTIONS

SBAs

Question 1

A 30-year-old woman at 26 weeks' gestation reports positive for group B streptococcus on the high vaginal swab culture. Choose the most appropriate course of action in this clinical situation.

A. Repeat the high vaginal swab at 37 weeks
B. Treat with oral antibiotics for one week
C. Advise that she will need intravenous antibiotics in labour
D. Treat with oral antibiotics after delivery for one week
E. Advise that, if untreated antenatally, it can lead to neonatal GBS septicaemia

Question 2

A 36-year-old HIV-positive woman on highly active anti-retroviral therapy (HAART) comes to see you after a positive pregnancy test. Which one of the following statements is not true with regard to her management?

A. Advise her to continue to take HAART throughout the pregnancy and postpartum.
B. Vaginal delivery is not recommended for women on HAART.
C. Screening for genital infections at booking and at 28 weeks' gestation.
D. Screening for Hepatitis C should be performed at booking.
E. Avoidance of breastfeeding reduces the risk of mother to child transmission.

Question 3

As part of the infectious diseases in pregnancy screening programme, all pregnant women are routinely offered screening for the following infections at their booking antenatal visit except which one?

A. Syphilis
B. Hepatitis C
C. HIV
D. Hepatitis B
E. Rubella

Question 4

Which one of the following factors does not influence the transmission of herpes to the fetus?

A. Mode of delivery
B. The use of fetal scalp electrodes
C. Type of maternal infection
D. Duration of rupture of membranes before delivery
E. Woman's partner with herpes virus infection

Question 5

A 28-year old woman had recurrent genital herpes at 28 and 33 weeks' gestation and was started on suppressive antiviral therapy. She is currently 39 weeks' gestation and presents in spontaneous labour with no active lesions. What is the recommended mode of delivery?

A. Forceps delivery
B. Ventouse delivery
C. Vaginal delivery
D. Emergency caesarean section
E. Both forceps and ventouse delivery

Question 6

A 32-year-old para 2 woman presented at 28 weeks' gestation with abdominal pain and uterine tightenings. She was reviewed in the antenatal day assessment unit. Abdominal examination revealed no obvious uterine activity and on speculum examination the cervix was closed and long. Her urine dipstick showed leucocytes 3+ and nitrates 3+. She was given antibiotics for a suspected urinary tract infection and was discharged home. Her past history revealed history of premature labour at 32 and 34 weeks' gestation. She subsequently presents with abdominal pain and urinary retention at 32 weeks' gestation. Abdominal examination reveals uterine contractions of 3 in 10 minutes and speculum examination revealed 6 cm dilated cervical os. Her vulva also reveals multiple painful vesicles suggestive of primary herpes infection. Choose one answer regarding how should she be delivered at this stage?

A. Forceps delivery
B. Ventouse delivery
C. Vaginal delivery
D. Emergency caesarean section
E. Both forceps and ventouse delivery

Question 7

A 32-year-old woman presented with painful vulva at 36 weeks' gestation. Clinical examination revealed multiple painful vesicles suggestive of genital herpes infection. She had a sexual health screening and was given oral acyclovir for 5 days. She was booked for elective caesarean section at 39 weeks' gestation. However, she presents at 38 weeks' in second stage and delivered vaginally within half an hour of admission to labour ward. The newborn baby develops neonatal herpes infection. What was the most likely mode of viral transmission to the fetus?

A. Blood borne
B. Direct contact with genital secretions
C. Transplacental
D. Postnatal transmission
E. Contact with maternal urine

Question 8

A 32-year-old para 2 woman presents to the antenatal day assessment unit with a 24-hour history of spontaneous rupture of membranes (SROM) at 40 weeks' gestation. She informs you that her first child was diagnosed with chickenpox 3 days ago. Examination reveals that she has vesicular lesions on the abdomen and her arms and legs suspicious of chickenpox. Speculum examination confirms SROM and not in labour at present. She does not remember if she had chickenpox during her childhood. A blood test for IgG antibody and IgM antibody for varicella infection is requested and a swab is taken from vesicular fluid for virology. The results come back 24 hours later and reveal positive for varicella IgG antibody but negative for IgM antibodies. The vesicular fluid is negative for varicella virology. How do you think she should be delivered at this stage?

A. Induction of labour if not in labour by now
B. Semi-elective caesarean section
C. Emergency caesarean section
D. Await spontaneous onset of delivery
E. Forceps delivery in second stage

Question 9

A 28-year-old Asian woman presents to her GP as she had come in close contact, 3 days previously, with her nephew, who had chickenpox. She is currently 32 weeks' pregnant and feels feverish. Examination does not reveal any rash on the body. The GP prescribes her paracetomol and warns her not to come in contact with other pregnant women. Her booking bloods are negative for varicella IgG antibodies. What should be her next step of management?

A. Oral acyclovir
B. Intravenous acyclovir
C. Intravenous varicella immunoglobulin (IVIG)
D. Emergency caesarean section
E. Oral vanciclovir

Question 10

A 29-year-old woman presents to her GP at 27 weeks' gestation with a rash on her trunk. She had developed this rash 10 hours previously and thought that she had developed a food allergy. On questioning she gives a history of coming in close contact, 3 days earlier, with her niece, who had developed chickenpox rash. General examination reveals rash typical of varicella or chickenpox. She is otherwise well. What is her next initial management following diagnosis of chickenpox rash?

A. Intravenous acyclovir
B. Oral gancyclovir for 7 days
C. Oral acyclovir for 7 days
D. Elective caesarean section at 39 weeks' gestation
E. Ultrasound scan for structural abnormalities in 5 weeks' time

Question 11

A 29-year-old Caucasian woman presented to her GP at 37 weeks' gestation with a chickenpox rash during winter season. She was prescribed oral acyclovir for 7 days but was warned to report back if unwell. Three days later she presents to the emergency department with severe shortness of breath. What is the likely diagnosis in her case?

A. Community-acquired pneumonia
B. Varicella zoster pneumonia
C. Exacerbation of her past tuberculosis
D. Drug-induced adult respiratory distress syndrome
E. Bronchitis due to allergy to pollen

Question 12

A 30-year-old woman comes to her GP for advice. She is a known epileptic and is currently on antiepileptic medication. She is planning to conceive in the next couple of months and would like to know the risks to her and the fetus if she gets pregnant. All of the following are true except which one?

A. Miscarriage rate is increased.
B. Seizure frequency can be increased by 10–30% during pregnancy.
C. The risk of aspiration during seizure and sudden unexpected death (SUDEP) may be increased.
D. The risk of congenital malformations in the fetus is increased by 2–3 fold.
E. All antiepileptic medications have the same teratogenic effects to the fetus.

EMQs

OPTIONS FOR QUESTIONS 1–3

A. Anti-retroviral therapy (ART) should be discontinued
B. ART can be continued
C. Allow vaginal delivery
D. Elective termination
E. CD4 count testing
F. IV acyclovir
G. Instrumental delivery
H. No treatment at present
I. Oral acyclovir
J. Offer elective caesarean section
K. Perform caesarean section
L. Commence highly active anti-retroviral therapy (HAART)

Instructions

Each of the clinical scenarios described below tests knowledge about the management of a pregnant woman with HIV. For each one select the single most appropriate management plan. Each option may be used once, more than once or not at all.

1. A 28-year-old woman with a positive HIV test, who was commenced on HAART for PMTCT (prevention of mother to child transmission), has delivered. She has a CD4 count of >500 cells/μL and there is concordance with her partner.
2. A 29-year-old woman taking HAART with a plasma viral load (VL) greater than 50 copies/ml is seen in the antenatal clinic at 36 weeks' gestation.
3. A 27-year-old woman is booked at 29 weeks' gestation and is tested HIV positive. She is currently asymptomatic.

OPTIONS FOR QUESTIONS 4–6

A. Nuchal translucency screening
B. Chorionic villus sampling (CVS)
C. Combined test
D. Amniocentesis
E. Quadruple test
F. Amniotomy
G. Triple test
H. Cell-free fetal DNA test
I. Amniodrainage
J. Cordocentesis

Instructions

For each clinical scenario below, choose the single most appropriate screening test from the above list of options. Each option may be used once, more than once or not at all.

4. A 28-year-old south Asian woman with a history of irregular menstrual cycles attends for her dating scan at 12 weeks' gestation and wishes to have the Down syndrome screening test. Based on the scan, she is dated as 15 weeks' gestation.
5. A 40-year-old woman, who teaches children with special needs, is 12 weeks into her first pregnancy and is very anxious about the risk of Down syndrome. She wishes to have a diagnostic test, but is not ready to take the risk of miscarriage associated with invasive testing.
6. A 38-year-old G2 para 1 at 13 weeks' gestation attends fetal medicine unit for counselling after the screen-positive combined screening results with a risk of 1:50 Down syndrome. She is very keen to have a definitive diagnosis and opts to have invasive testing.

OPTIONS FOR QUESTIONS 7–9

A. Await normal delivery
B. Immunoglobulin to mother
C. Deliver by caesarean section
D. Intravenous intrapartum antibiotics
E. Maternal vaccination
F. Neonatal vaccination
G. Postpartum maternal vaccination
H. Oral antibiotics to mother
 I. Immunoglobulin to the neonate
 J. No intervention needed

Instructions

For each clinical scenario below, choose the single most appropriate immediate plan of action from the above list of options. Each option may be used once, more than once or not at all.

7. A 30-year-old para 1 woman at 32 weeks' gestation seeks advice when her child is diagnosed with chickenpox and she is not sure whether she had chickenpox or not. She is non-immune for varicella zoster virus on blood test.

8. A 23-year-old nulliparous woman at 36 weeks' gestation attends the antenatal clinic after a recent diagnosis of genital herpes in the department of sexual health. She is on oral acyclovir and is anxious about the fetal effects and the mode of delivery.

9. A 26-year-old para 2 woman attends the antenatal clinic at 36 weeks' gestation. She was recently treated for sepsis secondary to urinary tract infection as an inpatient and was discharged on oral antibiotics. Midstream urine culture results showed group B streptococcus (GBS) infection. She recovered well and is asymptomatic.

OPTIONS FOR QUESTIONS 10–12

A. Folic acid 400 mcg supplementation
B. Aspirin 150 mg
C. Aspirin + low molecular weight heparin
D. Low molecular weight heparin (LMWH) antenatally and for 6 weeks postpartum
E. Folic acid 5 mg
F. Aspirin 75 mg
G. LMWH for 6 weeks postpartum
H. Aspirin 75 mg + folic acid 400 mcg
 I. Vitamin D supplementation
 J. Aspirin 75 mg + folic acid 5 mg

Instructions

For each clinical scenario below, choose the single most appropriate intervention from the above list of options. Each option may be used once, more than once or not at all.

10. A 42-year-old G2 para 1 woman attends the antenatal clinic after her dating scan at 12 weeks' gestation. She had early onset pre-eclampsia and fetal growth restriction requiring preterm delivery at 32 weeks' in her first pregnancy. She is concerned about the risk of pre-eclampsia in this pregnancy.
11. A 30-year-old nulliparous woman at 10 weeks' gestation attends the antenatal clinic. She is an insulin-dependent diabetic with good glycaemic control. She is taking multivitamins and concerned about the risks of diabetes in pregnancy.
12. A 32-year-old nulliparous woman attends her booking antenatal visit at 10 weeks' gestation. You have been asked to see this woman as she had a pulmonary embolism 2 years ago, while taking combined oral contraceptive pills.

OPTIONS FOR QUESTIONS 13–15

A. Ultrasound at 32 weeks
B. Reassurance
C. Ultrasound at 36 weeks
D. Refer to fetal medicine specialist
E. Uterine artery Dopplers
F. MRI pelvis
G. Abdominal and pelvic x-rays
H. Doppler ultrasound
 I. Immediate delivery
 J. Serial growth scans

Instructions

For each clinical scenario below, choose the single most appropriate advice from the above list of options. Each option may be used once, more than once or not at all.

13. A 30-year-old para 4 woman with four normal vaginal deliveries was referred for small for gestational age at 28 weeks. Her growth scan is normal with normal liquor and umbilical artery Dopplers. She is concerned as the report states that the fetus is in breech position.
14. A 20-year-old para 1 woman with a previous normal vaginal delivery has anomaly scan at 20 weeks' gestation which states that the placenta is posterior low. She is asymptomatic with no history of vaginal bleeding.
15. A 41-year-old para 2 woman with history of severe pre-eclampsia and fetal growth restriction in her first pregnancy attends the antenatal clinic at 22 weeks' gestation. Her anomaly scan is normal and she has been taking aspirin 75 mg from 12 weeks onwards.

MCQs

1. Antepartum haemorrhage (APH):
   A. Is bleeding from or into the genital tract before 20 weeks' gestation
   B. Is bleeding from or into the genital tract before 12 weeks' gestation
   C. Is bleeding from or into the genital tract after 28 weeks' gestation
   D. Is bleeding from or into the genital tract after 24 weeks' gestation
   E. Can be bleeding from the cervix after 24 weeks' gestation

2. Women with placental abruption can present with:
   A. Reduced fetal movements
   B. Presence of vaginal bleeding
   C. Absence of vaginal bleeding
   D. Neurogenic shock
   E. Severe abdominal pain

3. Clinical examination of a woman with placental abruption may reveal:
   A. Relaxed uterus
   B. Woody hard uterus
   C. Vaginal bleeding
   D. Anaemia proportion to visible vaginal blood loss
   E. Shock is out of proportion to the visible blood loss

4. The following are absolute indications for caesarean section:
   A. One previous caesarean section
   B. Two previous caesarean sections
   C. Placenta praevia
   D. Abruption placenta
   E. Active primary genital herpes

5. Absolute indications for caesarean section include:
   A. Maternal HIV infection
   B. HIV infection in the partner
   C. Presence of cervical polyp during pregnancy
   D. Cervical cancer during pregnancy
   E. Cervical intraepithelial neoplasia during pregnancy

6. The complications of placental abruption include:
   A. Chronic renal failure
   B. Chronic renal disease
   C. Acute renal failure
   D. Thrombocytopaenia
   E. Consumptive coagulopathy

7. The causes of APH include:
   A. Previous history of APH
   B. Cervical ectropion
   C. Multiple sexual partners
   D. Vasa praevia
   E. Velamentous insertion of the umbilical cord into the placenta

8. Placenta praevia:
   A. Is implantation of the embryo into the upper segment of uterus
   B. Is implantation of the embryo at the cornual region of uterus
   C. Can occur in women with a history of previous caesarean section
   D. Has been reported in women with previous history of dilatation and curettage
   E. Can lead to haemorrhagic shock and death of pregnant women

9. The following findings may be noted in a woman with placental abruption:
   A. Fetal distress
   B. Anaemia
   C. Bleeding from intravenous drip sites
   D. Blood-stained liquor
   E. Absence of the fetal heart beat

10. Grades of placenta praevia
    A. Grade 1: the placenta is implanted into the lower segment but encroaches on the cervical os
    B. Grade 2: the placenta is implanted into the lower segment but does not reach the margin of the cervical os
    C. Grade 3: the placenta covers the cervical os completely
    D. Grade 4: the placenta covers the cervical os partially
    E. Grade 5: the placenta is implanted in the cervical canal

11. Regarding herpes simplex virus (HSV) infection during pregnancy and labour:
    A. Recurrent herpes is associated with a very high risk of neonatal herpes.
    B. Paediatricians need to be alerted about the symptoms of maternal herpes in labour.
    C. Most perinatal infections are caused by herpes simplex type 2 virus.
    D. Primary genital herpes acquired within 6 weeks of delivery is associated with a significant risk of transmission to the fetus.
    E. Transplacental infection of the fetus is very common.

12. With regard to HSV infection:
    A. It is a RNA virus.
    B. Both type 1 and 2 HSV can cause genital infection in the pregnant woman.
    C. Both type 1 and 2 HSV from mother can be transmitted to the fetus at delivery.
    D. Herpes simplex virus is mainly transmitted to the fetus during delivery.
    E. Caesarean section is indicated in all women who give history of herpes simplex virus infection during pregnancy.

13. Regarding parvovirus infection:
    A. It is caused by parvovirus B19.
    B. It causes slapped-cheek syndrome in children.
    C. It may cause arthralgia in adults.
    D. It can cause severe fetal anaemia.
    E. It can cause immune hydrops in the fetus.

14. Parvovirus B19 infection:
    A. Is a DNA virus
    B. Is spread by sexual contact
    C. Has an incubation period of 10–14 days
    D. Can cause immune hydrops
    E. Can be diagnosed by maternal serology

15. With regard to primary genital herpes infection:
    A. Women should be referred to a sexual health clinic physician.
    B. Acyclovir can be safely used during the first trimester of pregnancy.
    C. The dose of acyclovir should be increased during pregnancy due to increased metabolism in the liver.
    D. All women with recurrent herpes should be offered type-specific antibody testing during pregnancy.
    E. Breastfeeding is contraindicated in women with primary herpes.

16. The following are either true or false with regard to chickenpox during pregnancy:
    A. A woman should be warned about the increased risk of miscarriage if she develops chickenpox within 20 weeks' gestation.
    B. A woman should be advised about the increased risk of fetal varicella syndrome if she develops chickenpox after 28 weeks' gestation.
    C. A woman should be advised that she will need an ultrasound scan 5 weeks later after infection to identify any structural abnormalities if she develops chickenpox before 28 weeks' gestation.
    D. A woman should be advised that the fetus can acquire the virus if she develops chickenpox later in the pregnancy and thereafter can remain dormant and can manifest later in life as shingles.
    E. A woman should be advised that she will have to terminate the pregnancy if she develops chickenpox after 28 weeks' gestation due to increased risk of fetus developing fetal varicella syndrome.

17. With regard to prevention of malaria in pregnancy and travel:
    A. Pregnant women do not need to worry about being exposed to malaria infection when visiting endemic areas.
    B. Pregnant women should avoid travel to endemic countries with malaria in view of inherent risks.
    C. Pregnant women should be advised about the possible symptoms of malaria if they are travelling to endemic countries.
    D. Pregnant women should be advised to take chemoprophylaxis against malaria if the trip to endemic countries is unavoidable.
    E. Mosquito-bite prevention measures don't prevent malaria in occurring during pregnancy when visiting endemic countries.

18. With regard to treatment of malaria during pregnancy:
    A. A 30-year-old African para 0 woman presents to the maternity day assessment unit at 36 weeks' gestation with fever, malaise and muscle pain. She gives a history of epilepsy and malaria during childhood. Peripheral blood smear shows *Plasmodium falciparum* (less than 2% parasitized red cells). She is otherwise stable. The drug of choice to treat her is primaquine.
    B. A 30-year-old black African para 1 woman presents to the maternity day assessment unit at 37 weeks' gestation with fever, malaise and muscle pain. She has been on holiday to Nigeria and returned to the UK one week ago. Peripheral blood film shows *Plasmodium vivax*. She is clinically stable and receives standard treatment for malaria and repeat peripheral blood film is normal. Four weeks later, she comes to the GP for advice as she is about to go on long holiday to Caribbean. The recommended chemoprophylactic drug for her is doxycycline.
    C. A 30-year-old African para 1 woman presents to the maternity day assessment unit at 36 weeks' gestation with fever, malaise and muscle pain. Her peripheral smear shows plasmodium ovale. She is otherwise stable. The drug of choice in her case is chloroquine.
    D. A 30-year-old African para 1 woman presents to the maternity day assessment unit at 34 weeks' gestation with symptoms of malaise, fever and headache and impaired consciousness. She has travelled to central Africa 3 weeks previously and has been back in the UK for a few days. Her peripheral blood film shows *P. falciparum* (more than 2% parasitized red blood cells) with severe thrombocytopenia. Her full blood count reveals haemoglobin (HB) of 6 gm% and arterial blood gas shows lactate of 4. The drug of choice in her case for treatment is chloroquine.
    E. A 30-year-old African para 1 woman presents to the maternity day assessment unit at 30 weeks' gestation with fever, malaise and myalgia. She visited Ghana 2 months ago. She is back in the UK and is asymptomatic. Peripheral blood smear shows *P. falciparum*. She vomits within half an hour of giving oral quinine. The GP advises that there is no need for further treatment.

19. With regard to iron and pregnancy:
    A. Requirements increase in pregnancy due to increase in erythropoiesis
    B. Daily requirement is around 6–7 mg
    C. Total average content in normal adult females is 2 gm
    D. Small intervals between pregnancies may increase the risk of deficiency
    E. At term, haemoglobin levels less than 10 gm% is due to deficiency rather than haemodilution of pregnancy

20. Regarding cardiac output during pregnancy:
    A. It starts to increase only at 20 weeks' gestation.
    B. The initial increase in the cardiac output is mainly due to an increase in the heart rate and decrease in peripheral vascular resistance.
    C. At 10–20 weeks' gestation, decreased cardiac output is mainly reflected by increase by stroke volume.
    D. It increases by 40% by 20–24 weeks' gestation.
    E. As pregnancy advances, cardiac output increases by 80% at term.

21. The effects of pregnancy on the gastrointestinal and genitourinary tract include:
    A. The appendix is displaced downwards into the pelvis.
    B. Gastric emptying time is delayed secondary to hormonal and mechanical factors.
    C. Bladder emptying time is delayed secondary to hormonal factors.
    D. Calyces, renal pelvis and ureters undergo marked dilatation.
    E. Progesterone may cause smooth-muscle relaxation and therefore increase the risk of vesico-ureteric reflux.

22. A 30-year-old woman is admitted to the antenatal ward at 32 weeks' gestation with mild pre-eclampsia.
    A. It is important to deliver her now in order to prevent her from developing severe pre-eclampsia.
    B. Her subsequent management during pregnancy depends on the severity of the disease.
    C. She may need anti-hypertensive medication if she develops moderate or severe pre-eclampsia.
    D. She may need at least twice-weekly pre-eclampsia blood tests.
    E. If a decision for delivery is made after 36 weeks of gestation, then administration of steroids for lung maturity will be necessary.

6

ANTENATAL CARE – ANSWERS

SBAs

Answer 1: C

Antenatal treatment with benzylpenicillin is not recommended if GBS is detected incidentally earlier in pregnancy, as approximately 21% of women are GBS carriers and it does not reduce the risk of colonization at delivery. Intravenous intrapartum antibiotics should be offered to women if GBS was detected on high vaginal swab in the current pregnancy or GBS bacteriuria in current pregnancy or previous history of neonatal GBS septicaemia, to minimize the risk of early onset neonatal GBS infection.

Further reading

RCOG Green-top guideline No. 36. *Early-onset group B streptococcal disease.* 2012. Available at: www.rcog.org.uk/womens-health/clinical-guidance /prevention-early-onset-neonatal-group-b-streptococcal-disease-green-top-36

Answer 2: B

In women who require HIV treatment for their own health, their prescribed HAART regimen should be continued throughout pregnancy and postpartum. At the booking antenatal visit, screening for syphilis, rubella, hepatitis B and also additional tests for hepatitis C, *Varicella zoster*, measles and toxoplasma should be performed. Screening for genital infections should be performed at booking and also at 28 weeks' gestation. Vaginal delivery may be offered to women on HAART with an undetectable viral load (<50 copies/ml).

Further reading

RCOG Green-top guideline No. 39. *HIV in pregnancy, management.* 2010. Available at: www.rcog.org.uk/womens-health/clinical-guidance /management-hiv-pregnancy-green-top-39

Answer 3: B

All pregnant women should be offered screening for hepatitis B, HIV, rubella and syphilis at booking visit. They should also have screening for asymptomatic bacteriuria by midstream urine culture in early pregnancy. Screening for hepatitis C, cytomegalovirus, toxoplasmosis, group B streptococcus, chlamydia, and asymptomatic bacterial vaginosis should not be offered as part of routine antenatal care.

Further reading

NICE clinical guideline No. 62. *Antenatal care*. 2008. Available at: www.nice.org.uk/nicemedia/pdf/CG062NICEguideline.pdf

Answer 4: E

The following factors influence the transmission of the virus to fetus:

- Type of maternal infection, whether primary or secondary herpes
- The presence of transplacental maternal neutralizing antibodies
- Duration of rupture of membranes before delivery
- The use of fetal scalp electrodes
- The use of fetal blood sampling
- The mode of delivery

Further reading

RCOG Green-top guideline No. 30. *Genital herpes in pregnancy, management*. 2007. Available at: www.rcog.org.uk/womens-health/clinical-guidance /management-genital-herpes-pregnancy-green-top-30

Answer 5: C

Recurrent herpes during antenatal period is not an indication for caesarean section as the risk of neonatal herpes is low (3%). The risk of transmission decreases to 1% if there are no visible lesions. Therefore, this woman could aim for a normal vaginal delivery. However, she should be thoroughly counselled about the risks and benefits of vaginal delivery versus caesarean section. During labour, one should carefully consider avoiding or delaying artificial rupture of membranes and invasive procedures on the fetus (e.g. fetal blood sampling or fetal scalp electrode for fetal monitoring).

Further reading

RCOG Green-top guideline No. 30. *Genital herpes in pregnancy, management.* 2007. Available at: www.rcog.org.uk/womens-health/clinical-guidance /management-genital-herpes-pregnancy-green-top-30

Answer 6: D

The highest chance of transmission to the fetus is when the primary infection occurs within 6 weeks of delivery (30–60%). Caesarean section is recommended for all women presenting with their first episode of genital herpes at the time of delivery, within 6 weeks of expected date of delivery (EDD) or with the onset of preterm delivery.

Further reading

RCOG Green-top guideline No. 30. *Genital herpes in pregnancy, management.* 2007. Available at: www.rcog.org.uk/womens-health/clinical-guidance /management-genital-herpes-pregnancy-green-top-30

Answer 7: B

Vertical transmission to the fetus mainly occurs at the time of delivery due to direct contact with the maternal genital secretions or through contact with the vesicles through skin breaks and rarely by transplacental and postnatal transmission. It can be reduced by suppressive maternal antiviral therapy during the last 4 weeks of pregnancy. Intravenous acyclovir given intrapartum to the mother and the neonate may reduce the risk of neonatal herpes in women who have their first episode of genital herpes at or within 6 weeks of delivery.

Further reading

RCOG Green-top guideline No. 30. *Genital herpes in pregnancy, management.* 2007. Available at: www.rcog.org.uk/womens-health/clinical-guidance /management-genital-herpes-pregnancy-green-top-30

Answer 8: A

The incidence of primary maternal infection with varicella zoster is 7 in 10,000 pregnancies (3 per 1000 reported in RCOG guideline). The risk of intrauterine fetal infection in pregnant women is 2% at 13–20 weeks' gestation.

More than 90% of women are already sero-positive (immune) due to previous clinical or sub-clinical disease in childhood (eight or nine out of every ten women in the UK turn out to be immune and have nothing to worry about).

If the woman has already had chickenpox in the past, then she is immune and therefore there is no need for concern. In this case, the woman was not sure whether she had chickenpox in the past. Therefore, she was tested for IgG. Her IgG antibody for varicella was positive and indicates that she is immune and so she can be reassured.

She is already 24 hours post SROM, therefore needs induction of labour.

Further reading

RCOG Green-top guideline No. 13. *Chickenpox in pregnancy*. September 2007. Available at: www.rcog.org.uk/womens-health/clinical-guidance /chickenpox-pregnancy-green-top-13

Answer 9: C

If the pregnant woman is not immune to VZV and she has had a significant exposure, she should be given VZIG as soon as possible. It may reduce the severity of the disease if she develops varicella or chickenpox but will not prevent her from developing chickenpox. VZIG is effective when given up to 10 days after contact. VZIG has no therapeutic benefit once chickenpox has developed.

Further reading

RCOG Green-top guideline No. 13. *Chickenpox in pregnancy*. September 2007. Available at: www.rcog.org.uk/womens-health/clinical-guidance /chickenpox-pregnancy-green-top-13

Answer 10: C

Pregnant women who develop a chickenpox rash should immediately contact their GP. The UK Advisory Group on chickenpox recommends that oral aciclovir be prescribed for pregnant women with chickenpox if they present within 24 hours of the onset of the rash and if they are more than 20 weeks' gestation. Acyclovir should be used cautiously before 20 weeks' gestation. Women should be informed of the potential risk and benefits of treatment with acyclovir. Oral acyclovir (800 mg five times a day for 7 days) reduces the duration of fever and symptomatology of varicella infection in immunocompetent adults if commenced within 24 hours of developing the rash, when compared with placebo.

A woman who comes in close contact with a person with chickenpox, or if she herself develops chickenpox, should avoid contact with susceptible individuals, including other pregnant women and neonates, until the lesions have crusted. Symptomatic treatment and hygienic measures are advised to prevent secondary bacterial infection of the lesions and septicaemia. However, if a secondary bacterial infection of the lesions develops, she will require antibiotics.

Further reading

RCOG Green-top guideline No. 13. *Chickenpox in pregnancy*. September 2007. Available at: www.rcog.org.uk/womens-health/clinical-guidance /chickenpox-pregnancy-green-top-13

Answer 11: B

A woman who develops a chickenpox rash should be warned to come to the emergency department or be referred immediately if she develops any of the following: chest symptoms, neurological symptoms, haemorrhagic rash or bleeding, a dense rash with or without mucosal lesions. If she is immunocompromised then she may need hospitalization and supportive care.

In this case the diagnosis is varicella pneumonia. The risk of varicella pneumonia in women who had chickenpox during pregnancy is around 10%. Mortality has been reported to be 20–45% in the pre-antiviral era but has been reduced to 3–14% with antiviral therapy and intensive care. The mortality in women with varicella pneumonia is due to associated complications, which include bacterial superinfection, adult respiratory distress syndrome, pneumonia and endotoxic shock. Therefore, appropriate treatment should be decided in consultation with a multidisciplinary team: obstetrician or fetal medicine specialist, virologist and neonatologist. Women hospitalized with varicella should be nursed in isolation from babies, potentially susceptible pregnant women or non-immune staff.

The neonatal death rate for varicella pneumonia is reported to be between 9 and 20%.

Further reading

RCOG Green-top guideline No. 13. *Chickenpox in pregnancy*. September 2007. Available at: www.rcog.org.uk/womens-health/clinical-guidance /chickenpox-pregnancy-green-top-13

Answer 12: E

Effect of Epilepsy and Antiepileptic Medication on Pregnancy and Fetus

Maternal Risks	Fetal Risks
Increased risk of miscarriage	2–3 fold increase in congenital malformations and stillbirths
She should be warned that the seizures may increase (10–30%), decrease or remain unchanged during pregnancy	Anti-folate action of the drugs are responsible for teratogenic action
Women with multiple seizure types are more likely to experience an increase in seizure frequency during pregnancy	Most antiepileptic medication causes fetal abnormalities
Risk of aspiration during seizure and increase in maternal mortality (also known as SUDEP)	Sodium valproate (up to 10%, especially neural tube defects) Phenytoin (4–5%) Carbamazepine (neural tube defects), Lamotrigene (2–3%) Limited information is available with regard to Levetiracetam, Topiramate, but currently seems reassuring.
Induction of liver enzymes and increase in drug dose requirements during pregnancy	The risk of the child developing epilepsy later in life is increased: 4–5% if either parent has epilepsy 15–20% if both parents have epilepsy 10% if there is an affected sibling

Further reading

Nelson-Piercy, C. *Handbook of Obstetric Medicine*. 4th ed. London: Informa Healthcare; 2010.

EMQs

Answers 1–3

1. A
ART should be discontinued in all women who commenced HAART for prevention of mother-to-child transmission (MTCT) with a CD4 count of >500 cells/µl.

ART should be continued postpartum in all women who commenced HAART for MTCT:

- with a CD4 count of between 350 and 500 cells/µL during pregnancy who are coinfected with hepatitis B virus (HBV) or hepatitis C virus (HCV);
- with history of an AIDS-defining illness; or
- with a CD4 count of <350 cells/µL.

2. J
Delivery by elective caesarean section at 38 weeks to prevent labour and/or ruptured membranes is recommended for:

- women taking HAART who have a plasma viral load greater than 50 copies/ml;
- women taking ZDV monotherapy as an alternative to HAART; or
- women with HIV and hepatitis C virus coinfection.

Consider administration of glucocorticoids (steroids) pre-caesarean section when <39 weeks.

3. L
A woman who presents after 28 weeks should commence HAART without delay. If the VL is unknown or >100,000 HIV RNA copies/mL a three- or four-drug regimen is recommended. It is suggested that intravenous zidovudine be infused for the duration of labour and delivery.

Further reading

RCOG Green-top guideline No. 39. *Management of HIV in pregnancy*. 2010. Available at: www.rcog.org.uk/womens-health/clinical-guidance/management-hiv-pregnancy-green-top-39

British HIV Association guidelines. *Management of HIV infection in pregnant women*. 2012. Available at: www.bhiva.org/PregnantWomen2012.aspx.

Answers 4–6

4. E

As the above patient is already 15 weeks, the quadruple test is the effective serum screening test offered between 15+0 and 20+0 weeks' gestation.

Further reading

NICE clinical guideline 62. *Antenatal care*. 2010. Available at: www.nice.org.uk /nicemedia/live/11947/40115/40115.pdf

5. H

Harmony test or maternal serum for cell-free fetal DNA is a non-invasive test for testing fetal aneuploidy, not yet routinely offered in NHS.

Further reading

Benn P, Cuckle H, Pergament E. Non-invasive prenatal testing for aneuploidy: current status and future prospects. *Ultrasound Obstet Gynaecol*. 2013; 42: 15–33.

6. B

CVS is usually performed between 11+0 and 13+6 weeks' gestation and involves aspiration or biopsy of placental villi. Amniocentesis is performed to obtain amniotic fluid from 15 weeks onwards.

Further reading

RCOG Green-top guideline No. 8. *Amniocentesis and chorionic villus sampling*. 2010. Available at: www.rcog.org.uk/files/rcog-corp/GT8Amniocentesis0111.pdf

Answers 7–9

7. B

If the pregnant woman is not immune and she has had a significant exposure to chickenpox, she should be given varicella zoster immunoglobulin (VZIG) as soon as possible. VZIG is effective when given up to 10 days after contact.

Further reading

RCOG Green-top guideline No. 13. *Chickenpox in pregnancy*. 2007. Available at: www.rcog.org.uk/files/rcog-corp/uploaded-files /GT13ChickenpoxinPregnancy2007.pdf

8. C

Caesarean section is recommended to all women with primary episode of herpes simplex virus (HSV) infection at the time of delivery or within 6 weeks of expected date of delivery.

Further reading

RCOG Green-top guideline No. 30. *Management of genital herpes in pregnancy.* 2007. Available at: www.rcog.org.uk/files/rcog-corp/uploaded-files /GT30GenitalHerpes2007.pdf

9. D

Intrapartum intravenous antibiotic prophylaxis should be offered to women with GBS bacteriuria or GBS detected on vaginal swab in the current pregnancy and to women with a previous baby with neonatal GBS sepsis.

Further reading

RCOG Green-top guideline No. 36. *Prevention of early-onset neonatal group B streptococcal disease.* 2012. Available at: www.rcog.org.uk/files/rcog-corp /GTG36_GBS.pdf

Answers 10–12

10. F

Further reading

NICE clinical guideline 107. *Hypertension in pregnancy: The management of hypertensive disorders during pregnancy.* 2011. Available at: www.nice.org.uk /nicemedia/live/13098/50418/50418.pdf

11. J

Women with diabetes are at high risk for pre-eclampsia. Aspirin 75 mg daily from 12 weeks till birth of the baby is recommended to minimize the risk. Folic acid 5 mg/day till 12 weeks, gestation is recommended to reduce the risk of the baby developing neural tube defects.

Further reading

NICE clinical guideline 63. *Diabetes in pregnancy: Management of diabetes and its complications from pre-conception to the postnatal period.* 2008. Available at: www.nice.org.uk/nicemedia/pdf/cg063guidance.pdf

12. D

Antenatal thromboprophylaxis with LMWH should begin as early as possible and continue for 6 weeks postpartum in women who are at very high risk for developing VTE during pregnancy.

Antenatal thromboprophylaxis with LMWH should be offered to women who have the following:

- a previous recurrent VTE;
- a previous unprovoked or oestrogen or pregnancy-related VTE;
- a previous VTE and a history of VTE in a first-degree relative; or
- a documented thrombophilia.

Further reading

RCOG Green-top guideline No. 37a. *Thrombosis and embolism during pregnancy and the puerperium, reducing the risk.* 2009. Available at: www.rcog.org.uk /womens-health/clinical-guidance/reducing-risk-of-thrombosis-greentop37a

Answers 13–15

13. B

The incidence of breech presentation decreases from about 20% at 28 weeks' gestation to 3–4% at term, as most babies turn spontaneously to the cephalic presentation. The lie of her baby is likely to be affected by her multiparity.

Further reading

RCOG Green-top guideline No. 20b. *The management of breech presentation.* Available at: www.rcog.org.uk/files/rcog-corp/GtG%20no%2020b%20 Breech%20presentation.pdf

14. C

In all asymptomatic women with suspected placenta previa, a repeat ultrasound to assess placental site can be left until 36 weeks' gestation unless indicated earlier to measure the growth of the fetus or for vaginal bleeding.

Further reading

RCOG Green-top guideline No. 27. *Placenta praevia, placenta praevia accreta and vasa praevia: diagnosis and management.* 2011. Available at: www.rcog.org.uk /files/rcog-corp/GTG27PlacentaPraeviaJanuary2011.pdf

15. J

Serial growth scans including umbilical artery Dopplers from 26–28 weeks onwards should be arranged in view of the presence of major risk factors like age >40 yrs, previous pre-eclampsia and fetal growth restriction.

Further reading

RCOG Green-top guideline No. 31. *The investigation and management of the small-for-gestational-age fetus.* Available at: www.rcog.org.uk/files /rcog-corp/22.3.13GTG31SGA_ExecSum.pdf

MCQs

1A: False
1B: False
1C: True
1D: True
1E: True

APH is defined as bleeding from or into the genital tract after 24 weeks' gestation and before delivery.

The incidence of APH is 3–5% of pregnancies. It is associated with major morbidity and mortality for both mother and the fetus. The incidence increases with increasing age and parity.

Further reading

RCOG Green-top guideline No. 27. *Placenta praevia, placenta praevia accreta and vasa praevia: diagnosis and management.* 2011. Available at: www.rcog.org.uk /files/rcog-corp/GTG27PlacentaPraeviaJanuary2011.pdf

2A: True
2B: True
2C: True
2D: False
2E: True

Clinical presentation of placental abruption include:

- Vaginal bleeding: may be revealed or concealed or both
    1. Revealed: in this situation the woman presents with vaginal bleeding. The blood may dissect under the membranes and track down between the uterine wall and the membranes to reach the cervix and the vagina.
    2. Concealed: in this situation the woman does not present with vaginal bleeding but may present with other symptoms, such as severe abdominal pain and shock. In this situation the bleeding is mainly retro-placental even with complete detachment of the placenta. Therefore, the woman does not present with vaginal bleeding but has other symptoms (severe abdominal pain and signs of shock). The amount of vaginal bleeding does not exactly correlate either to the total amount of blood loss or to the extent of anaemia clinically or haematologically. The anaemia is usually out of proportion to the visible blood loss.
    3. Both revealed and concealed: there is vaginal bleeding but this does not truly reflect the amount of blood loss or anaemia because the bleeding is also retro-placental.
    4. Bleeding into the uterine muscle or Couvelaire uterus: if there is an increase in intrauterine pressure due to excessive bleeding, the blood can seep through in between the uterine muscle fibres (myometrium). This leads to an inflammatory response and tonic uterine contraction. It leaves a different colour (bruised) to the uterus due to extravasation of the blood within the myometrium. This is named the Couvelaire uterus.

- Abdominal pain (50%): is usually severe and constant pain, rather than regularly spaced uterine contraction pain
- Backache: women with posterior placenta can have backache
- Reduced fetal movements: with major retroplacental bleed they may have reduced or lack of fetal movements
- Shock: with extreme blood loss they may present with shock

Further reading

Collins S, Arulkumaran S, et al. *Oxford Handbook of Obstetrics & Gynaecology*. 3rd ed. Oxford: Oxford University Press; 2013.

3A: False
3B: True
3C: True
3D: False
3E: True

Clinical signs of placental abruption include:

- Uterus tense and tender (described as woody hard)
- Anaemia is out of proportion to the blood loss
- Shock is out of proportion to the blood loss
- Vaginal bleeding
- Blood stained liquor
- Bleeding from other sites when in disseminated intravascular coagulation (DIC) (e.g. cannula site, haematuria, nose bleed and bruising)
- Fetal distress and death (CTG abnormality)
- Absence of fetal heart beat on sonicaid
- May find difficulty in palpating the fetal parts
- Premature labour
- Hypertension
- Sometimes pain and bleeding may not be present

Further reading

Collins S, Arulkumaran S, et al. *Oxford Handbook of Obstetrics & Gynaecology*. 3rd ed. Oxford: Oxford University Press; 2013.

4A: False
4B: False
4C: False – The incidence of placenta praevia is 20% in second trimester but falls to 2–3% by term. This is because the placenta appears to move upwards due to differential growth of the uterine lower segment below it as the pregnancy advances. Therefore, a repeat ultrasound scan at 32–34 weeks' gestation is indicated to determine the location of the placenta. The diagnosis of placenta praevia is not an absolute indication for caesarean section as the delivery method depends on the grade of placenta praevia. Grade 1 can be considered for vaginal delivery, but most grade 2, grade 3 and grade 4 should be delivered by caesarean section.

4D: False

4E: True – When there is active primary genital herpes, caesarean section is recommended to reduce the risk of neonatal transmission at delivery.

Further reading

RCOG Green-top guideline No. 27. *Placenta praevia, placenta praevia accreta and vasa praevia: diagnosis and management*. 2011. Available at: www.rcog.org.uk /files/rcog-corp/GTG27PlacentaPraeviaJanuary2011.pdf

5A: False – Caesarean section along with retroviral therapy reduces the vertical transmission to less than 1% in the neonate. Therefore, caesarean section is recommended. However, if the viral load is less than 50 copies, vaginal delivery can be considered in these women with AZT coverage in labour.
5B: False
5C: False
5D: True
5E: False

Further reading

Collins S, Arulkumaran S, et al. *Oxford Handbook of Obstetrics & Gynaecology*. 3rd ed. Oxford: Oxford University Press; 2013.

6A: False
6B: False
6C: True
6D: True
6E: True – DIC

The incidence of placental abruption is less than 1% of pregnancies. It is defined as premature separation of the normally situated placenta. Bleeding occurs due to separation of the placenta before the delivery of the fetus. The bleeding starts in the decidua basalis and, with increasing bleeding, the placenta begins to separate from its attachment to the uterine wall. If the bleeding is minimal the separation of the placenta may be partial and self-limiting. But if the bleeding is severe, it may lead to complete detachment of the placenta, which may then lead to fetal hypoxia and fetal death.

Complications of placental abruption include:

- Haemorrhagic shock
- Massive postpartum haemorrhage
- Multi-organ failure due to massive haemorrhage
- Maternal death
- Fetal hypoxia and death
- Severe fetal anaemia requiring blood transfusion at birth
- Feto-maternal haemorrhage and sensitization in a woman who is Rhesus negative
- Couvelaire uterus: may impair uterine contractility and contribute to PPH
- Sheehan's syndrome due to massive PPH and pituitary necrosis
- Premature delivery

Further reading

Collins S, Arulkumaran S, et al. *Oxford Handbook of Obstetrics & Gynaecology.* 3rd ed. Oxford: Oxford University Press; 2013.

7A: False
7B: True
7C: False
7D: True
7E: True

Causes and differential diagnosis of APH include:

- Placental causes: placenta praevia, placental abruption and bleeding from placental margin
- Local causes: cervical (polyp, ectropion and carcinoma), vaginal and vulval lesions
- Vasa praevia (rare)
- Unknown
- Abruption is associated with placenta praevia in 10% of the cases

Further reading

RCOG Green-top guideline No. 27. *Placenta praevia, placenta praevia accreta and vasa praevia: diagnosis and management.* 2011. Available at: www.rcog.org.uk /files/rcog-corp/GTG27PlacentaPraeviaJanuary2011.pdf

8A: False – Is implantation of the embryo on the lower segment
8B: False
8C: True
8D: True
8E: True

Placenta praevia is when the placenta is partially or wholly implanted into the lower uterine segment. The incidence of placenta praevia is 20% at the end of second trimester and falls to 2–3% at term.

Further reading

Collins S, Arulkumaran S, et al. *Oxford Handbook of Obstetrics & Gynaecology.* 3rd ed. Oxford: Oxford University Press; 2013.

9A: True
9B: True
9C: True
9D: True
9E: True

Further reading

RCOG Green-top guideline No. 63. *Antepartum haemorrhage.* 2011. Available at: www.rcog.org.uk/womens-health/clinical-guidance /antepartum-haemorrhage-green-top-63

10A: False
10B: False
10C: False
10D: False
10E: False – there is no grade 5

Grades of placenta praevia (1–4)

Grade 1: the placenta is implanted into the lower segment but does not encroach on the cervical os

Grade 2: the placenta is implanted into the lower segment but reaches the margin of the cervical os

Grade 3: the placenta covers the cervical os partially

Grade 4: the placenta covers the cervical os completely

Further reading

RCOG Green-top guideline No. 63. *Antepartum haemorrhage.* 2011. Available at: www.rcog.org.uk/womens-health/clinical-guidance/antepartum-haemorrhage-green-top-63

RCOG Green-top guideline No. 27. *Placenta praevia, placenta praevia accreta and vasa praevia: diagnosis and management.* 2011. Available at: www.rcog.org.uk/files/rcog-corp/GTG27PlacentaPraeviaJanuary2011.pdf

Collins S, Arulkumaran S, et al. *Oxford Handbook of Obstetrics & Gynaecology.* 3rd ed. Oxford: Oxford University Press; 2013.

11A: False – The risk of transmission to the fetus is much less (3%) with recurrent herpes
11B: True
11C: True
11D: True
11E: False – Transplacental infection of the fetus is rare

Further reading

RCOG Green-top guideline No. 30. *Genital herpes in pregnancy, management.* 2007. Available at: http://www.rcog.org.uk/womens-health/clinical-guidance/management-genital-herpes-pregnancy-green-top-30

12A: False – It is a DNA virus
12B: True
12C: True
12D: True
12E: False – The risk of fetal transmission is significantly higher if the mother acquires primary herpes infection at or within 6 weeks of delivery. If this is the case, caesarean section is recommended for delivery.

Genital herpes is caused by HSV, which is a DNA virus. There are two types of HSV: type 1 and type 2. Type 1 mainly causes oculo-oral lesions and type 2 mainly causes genital lesions. However, type 1 virus can cause both oculo-oral and genital lesions. Primary infection with HSV type 2 is typically associated with painful genital ulceration. Swabs from vesicle fluid can also be taken for culture. Treatment of genital lesions is mainly supportive (pain relief and treatment of secondary infection). Oral acyclovir (200 mg five times for 5 days) is used in cases of primary genital HSV and this may reduce the severity and shorten the duration of symptoms.

HSV can cause fetal infection in the perinatal period and these are mainly due to type 2 HSV. The risk of transmission to the fetus increases significantly if the infection in the mother is a primary infection (i.e. first-time genital HSV infection). HSV is transmitted to the fetus during its passage through the birth canal. The risk of transmission to the fetus or neonate is much lower (around 3%) with recurrent herpes due to transfer of passive immunity from the mother.

Caesarean section is recommended in women if the primary genital HSV infection is within 6 weeks of labour or active lesions are visible at the time of labour (there is no benefit of caesarean section if the membranes have ruptured for more than 4 hours). Women with recurrent herpes can have vaginal delivery as the risk to fetus is low and therefore not considered an indication for delivery by caesarean section. Paediatricians need to be informed as it can cause serious infections in the neonate including disseminated disease (mortality 70–80%). It can cause life-threatening pneumonia and encephalitis (mortality >90%) in the newborn with long-term sequelae.

Further reading

RCOG Green-top guideline No. 30. *Genital herpes in pregnancy, management.* 2007. Available at: http://www.rcog.org.uk/womens-health/clinical-guidance/management-genital-herpes-pregnancy-green-top-30

13A: True
13B: True
13C: True
13D: True
13E: False

Human parvovirus B19 is a DNA virus that belongs to the family Parvoviridae. The incubation period is 4–14 days. Women are infectious 3–10 days post exposure or until the appearance of the rash. The virus is spread by infected respiratory droplets.

About 50% of the pregnant women are immune to this virus and therefore protected. Pregnant women who acquire this infection are often asymptomatic. Women who are symptomatic may present with a non-specific illness such as rash (erythema infectiosum), fever, fatigue, lymphadenopathy and arthralgia (affects 80% of adults and 10% of children). In children it can cause mild infection (e.g. slapped-cheek syndrome or 5th disease).

Further reading

Collins S, Arulkumaran S, et al. *Oxford Handbook of Obstetrics & Gynaecology*. 3rd ed. Oxford: Oxford University Press; 2013.

14A: True
14B: False – It is spread by respiratory droplets
14C: True
14D: False – It causes non-immune hydrops
14E: True

Parvovirus B19 infection and fetal complications

Fetal effects include:

- miscarriage;
- severe anaemia;
- non-immune hydrops; and
- fetal cardiac failure and intrauterine death.

Fetal transmission of infection can occur in all trimesters. The risk of fetal loss is around 10% if the mother is positive for IgM and these mostly occur 4–6 weeks from the onset of maternal symptoms or infection. Non-immune hydrops occurs in 3% with a fatality rate of 50%. Spontaneous resolution is not uncommon. Generally, there are no long-term sequelae following resolution of the infection.

Diagnosis

The diagnosis is made by taking paired maternal serum samples and also by using PCR parvovirus genome.

Interpretation of serology results

- The presence of IgM antibodies indicates recent infection.
- The absence of both IgM and IgG antibodies suggest no previous infection but the person is susceptible to infection.
- The presence of only parvovirus B19 IgG indicates previous infection at least 4 months ago.
- When both parvovirus B19 IgM and IgG antibodies are present, it indicates recent infection between 7 days to 4 months.

Management of women infected with parvovirus infection

- The mother can be treated symptomatically.
- Women who are non-immune and currently not infected should be advised to avoid contact with other people with parvovirus B19 infection while they are pregnant.
- Termination of pregnancy should be discussed if infection occurs in early pregnancy.
- Arrange weekly serial ultrasound scans after 4 weeks of maternal exposure or infection in view of the risk of severe fetal anaemia and hydrops.

- If the ultrasound shows signs of hydrops or fetal anaemia, cord blood sampling and in-utero blood transfusion is indicated.
- Fetal growth scans should be arranged following resolution of hydrops.
- If the pregnancy is advanced, delivery should be considered.

Further reading

Collins S, Arulkumaran S, et al. *Oxford Handbook of Obstetrics & Gynaecology*. 3rd ed. Oxford: Oxford University Press; 2013.

15A: True – Women should be referred to genitourinary clinic to screen for other STDs.
15B: False – There is no definite evidence of teratogenicity; however, one should use acyclovir with caution before 20 weeks' gestation.
15C: False – Dose adjustment is not necessary during pregnancy.
15D: False – Type-specific HSV testing is offered to women who develop primary herpes (or first episode of HSV infection) in the third trimester of pregnancy to determine if it is primary infection or not. If the primary infection occurs within 6 weeks of the expected date of delivery or at the time of labour, a caesarean section should be recommended. However, if vaginal delivery is opted for by the woman, measures should be taken to reduce the risk of transmission of HSV infection to the fetus. These include avoiding artificial rupture of membranes, fetal blood sampling and fetal scalp electrode insertion. Also consider administering intravenous acyclovir to both mother and neonate.
15E: False – Breastfeeding is not contraindicated during postnatal period.

Further reading

RCOG Green-top guideline No. 30. *Genital herpes in pregnancy, management*. 2007. Available at: www.rcog.org.uk/womens-health/clinical-guidance /management-genital-herpes-pregnancy-green-top-30

16A: False – Women should be advised that the risk of spontaneous miscarriage does not appear to be increased if chickenpox occurs in the first trimester.
16B: False – If the pregnant woman develops varicella or shows serological conversion in the first 28 weeks of pregnancy, she has a small risk of fetal varicella syndrome (2%) and will need to be informed of the implications.
16C: True – Referral to a fetal medicine specialist should be considered at 16–20 weeks if the woman presents before 20 weeks' gestation or 5 weeks after infection for discussion and detailed ultrasound examination. Amniocentesis is not routinely advised because the risk of fetal varicella syndrome is so low, even when amniotic fluid is positive for varicella zoster virus (VZV) DNA. The risks versus benefits of the procedure should be discussed with the woman in conjunction with the findings on ultrasound examination.
16D: True – Once it is acquired, the VZV remains dormant in the body and manifests later in life as shingles.
16E: False – The risk of fetal varicella syndrome is negligible if the woman develops chickenpox after 28 weeks' gestation. The fetus may acquire the virus

but may not manifest until later in life after birth as shingles. There is no need to terminate the pregnancy.

Further reading

RCOG Green-top guideline No. 13. *Chickenpox in pregnancy*. 2007.
Available at: www.rcog.org.uk/files/rcog-corp/uploaded-files
/GT13ChickenpoxinPregnancy2007.pdf

17A: False
17B: True
17C: True
17D: True
17E: False

Pregnant women in UK who are non-immune are at risk of certain consequences due to malaria, which include:

- Susceptibility to infection
- Severe malaria or cerebral malaria
- Miscarriage, stillbirth and prematurity
- Increased maternal and fetal mortality
- May lead to reduction in the birth weight of fetus

If the trip to endemic countries is unavoidable the pregnant woman should be given the following advice, which can be summarized under the acronym ABCD.

- A: awareness of the risk of malaria as mentioned above and risk of acquiring malaria when visiting certain countries including Oceania (Papua New Guinea, Papua, Solomon Islands and Vanuatu) 1:20, Sub-Saharan Africa 1:50, Indian subcontinent 1:500, Southeast Asia 1:500, South America 1:2500, Central America and the Caribbean 1:10,000.
- B: bite prevention measures when travelling to endemic countries including skin repellents, knock-down mosquito sprays, insecticide-treated bed nets, clothing and room protection.
- C: chemoprophylaxis against malaria. Women should be advised that prophylaxis is not 100% effective. They should choose an alternative destination for travel unless unavoidable and also should seek advice from a specialist with current experience of malaria. The choice of drug chemoprophylaxis in pregnant women depends on the resistance of *Plasmodium falciparum* and *Plasmodium vivax* to chloroquine and trimester of pregnancy.
  - The drugs that can be used for chemoprophylaxis include:
    - Chloroquine and proguanil, which are safe and can be used in chloroquine-sensitive areas. They are not recommended in chloroquine-resistant areas.
    - Mefloquine (5 mg/kg once a week) is the recommended drug of choice for prophylaxis in the second and third trimester. The use of this drug in first trimester should be considered only after discussion with a specialist.

— Atovaquone and proguanil (Malarone) may be considered for prophylaxis in the second and third trimesters but it is not recommended, owing to insufficient data on its safety in pregnancy.
— Doxycycline and primaquine are contraindicated as chemoprophylaxis in pregnant women.

- D: diagnosis and treatment, which must be prompt when symptoms occur. Women should be advised about the symptoms (flu-like illness and raised temperature) and treated as emergency if malaria is suspected. Antipyretics should be used liberally to control temperature. Quinine (300 mg tablets, two tablets three times a day for 7 days) and clindamycin (150 mg capsules, three capsules three times a day for 5–7 days) are recommended in the UK. If a dose is vomited within 30 minutes, the full dose should be repeated and if the dose is vomited after 30–60 minutes, half the dose should be repeated. The treatment should be finished and mefloquine should be commenced 1 week after the last treatment dose.

Further reading

RCOG Green-top guideline No. 54A. *Malaria in pregnancy prevention*. 2010. Available at: www.rcog.org.uk/prevention-malaria-pregnancy-green-top-54a

18A: False – In this case, since the woman is stable, she has uncomplicated falciparum malaria. Uncomplicated malaria in the UK is defined as fewer than 2% parasitized red blood cells in a woman with no signs of severity and no complicating features.

The treatment in such cases includes:

- oral quinine 600 mg 8 hourly and oral clindamycin 450 mg 8 hourly for 7 days (can be given together); or
- riamet 4 tablets/dose for weight >35 kg, twice daily for 3 days (with fat); or
- atovaquone-proguanil (Malarone) 4 standard tablets daily for 3 days.

18B: False – Doxycycline is contraindicated during pregnancy. It can affect bone growth and cause permanent discoloration of the teeth in fetus when given in the 3rd trimester. Anecdotal case reports of congenital cataract have also been reported. Primaquine can cause haemolysis, particularly in G6PD deficiency.

18C: True – The treatment of non-falciparum malaria (*P. vivax, P. ovale, P. malariae)* is oral chloroquine (base) 600 mg followed by 300 mg 6 hours later, followed by 300 mg on day 2 and again on day 3.

18D: False – Malaria can present with non-specific flu-like illness. The symptoms include headache, fever with chills, nausea, vomiting, diarrhoea, coughing and general malaise. The signs of malaria can be raised temperature, splenomegaly, jaundice, pallor, sweating and respiratory distress.

The features of complicated or severe malaria include prostration, impaired consciousness, respiratory distress (ARDS), pulmonary oedema, convulsions, collapse, abnormal bleeding, DIC, jaundice, haemoglobinuria and algid malaria (a rare complication of falciparum malaria involving the gut where patient presents with cold, clammy skin, hypotension and diarrhoea).

The laboratory findings include severe anaemia, thrombocytopenia, hypoglycaemia, acidosis, renal impairment, hyperlactataemia, hyperparasitaemia and meningitis.

Microscopic diagnosis allows species identification and estimation of parasitaemia. Pregnant women with 2% or more parasitized red blood cells are at higher risk of developing severe malaria and should be treated with the severe malaria protocol.

In such women RCOG recommends:

- Admission of women with uncomplicated malaria to hospital
- Admission of women with complicated malaria to intensive care unit
- Intravenous artesunate as first line for the treatment of severe falciparum malaria
- Intravenous quinine if artesunate is not available
- Use of quinine and clindamycin to treat uncomplicated *P. falciparum* (or mixed, such as *P. falciparum* and *P. vivax*)
- Use of chloroquine to treat *P. vivax*, *P. ovale* or *P. Malariae*
- Primaquine use avoided in pregnancy
- Involving infectious disease specialists, especially for severe and recurrent cases
- If vomiting persists, oral therapy should be stopped and intravenous therapy should be instituted
- Treatment of the fever with antipyretics
- Screening for anaemia and treat appropriately
- Arranging follow up to ensure detection of relapse

18E: False – Vomiting is a known adverse effect of quinine and is associated with malarial treatment failure. Use antiemetic if the patient vomits and repeat the antimalarial medication. If the vomiting is persistent even after administration of antiemetics, then parenteral therapy is recommended.

Uncomplicated falciparum malaria with vomiting

- Quinine 10 mg/kg dose IV in 5% dextrose over 4 hours then every 8 hours plus IV clindamycin 450 mg every 8 hours
- Once the patient stops vomiting she can be switched to oral quinine 600 mg 3 times a day to complete 5–7 days and oral clindamycin can, if needed, be switched to 450 mg 3 times a day 7 days

Further reading

RCOG Green-top guideline No. 54b. *Diagnosis and treatment of malaria in pregnancy*. 2010. Available at: www.rcog.org.uk /diagnosis-and-treatment-malaria-pregnancy-green-top-54b

19A: True
19B: True
19C: True
19D: True
19E: True

Physiological anaemia of pregnancy

- Plasma volume increases by 50% beginning from the 6th week of pregnancy.
- Red blood cell (TBC) mass increases by 20–35% beginning from the 12th week of pregnancy.
- Plasma volume increase is more than RBC volume and therefore leads to haemodilution.
- Despite increase in the RBC mass, there is a fall in haemoglobin and haematocrit levels. This is known as physiological anaemia of pregnancy.
- Total iron requirement for normal pregnancy is around 1000 mg (200 mg is excreted, 300 mg is transferred to the fetus and 500 mg is iron requirements of the mother). The requirement is 1 mg/day in first trimester, 4–5 mg/day in second trimester and more than 6 mg in third trimester.

Further reading

Collins S, Arulkumaran S, et al. *Oxford Handbook of Obstetrics & Gynaecology.* 3rd ed. Oxford: Oxford University Press; 2013.

20A: False – Cardiac output starts to increase from as early as 5 weeks.
20B: True – Increase in cardiac output during early pregnancy is due to an increase in the heart rate and also a decrease in the peripheral vascular resistance.
20C: False – The increase in plasma volume or preload increases the stroke volume. This increase in stroke volume is responsible for increase in cardiac output by 10–20 weeks' gestation.
20D: True
20E: False – The heart rate continues to increase as pregnancy advances, while stroke volume falls close to normal levels. This is why cardiac output levels fall almost to near normal non-pregnant values at term.

Further reading

Collins S, Arulkumaran S, et al. *Oxford Handbook of Obstetrics & Gynaecology.* 3rd ed. Oxford: Oxford University Press; 2013.

21A: False – The appendix is usually displaced upwards higher up near the flank due to gravid uterus.
21B: True – Intestinal transit time is delayed secondary to hormonal and mechanical factors.
21C: False
21D: True
21E: True

Changes in the gastrointestinal and genitourinary tract during pregnancy

- Gravid uterus displaces stomach and intestines
- Vascular swelling of the gums
- Haemorrhoids occur due to an increase in pressure in the venous system

- Renal plasma flow and glomerular filtration (GFR) increases 40% by midgestation.
- Elevated GFR is reflected in the lower serum creatinine and blood urea nitrogen.
- Protein in the urine is generally not evident.

Further reading

Collins S, Arulkumaran S, et al. *Oxford Handbook of Obstetrics & Gynaecology.*
    3rd ed. Oxford: Oxford University Press; 2013.

22A: False – The aim of management is to prolong pregnancy as long as possible in mild pre-eclampsia.
22B: True
22C: True
22D: True
22E: False

Pre-eclampsia is defined as the presence of raised blood pressure (140/90 or more) after 20 weeks' gestation with significant proteinuria with or without oedema. It is a common complication of pregnancy that is associated with significant maternal and perinatal morbidity and mortality.

It can be graded as mild, moderate or severe. The aim is to prolong pregnancy as much as possible. Mild disease can be treated conservatively (observation, regular blood tests and antihypertensives). Moderate pre-eclampsia may need admission for observation, antihypertensives, regular blood tests (FBC, U&Es, uric acid, LFTs, coagulation profile) and 24-hour urine collection to quantify urinary protein. Severe pre-eclampsia would need delivery after stabilization of the woman (control of blood pressure, prevention of seizures and delivery of the fetus). The prevention of eclampsia is by the administration of magnesium sulphate.

Pre-eclampsia affects 3% of pregnant women and out of these only 10% will develop severe pre-eclampsia. If a woman has a history of pre-eclampsia, giving aspirin (75 mg daily) would reduce the risk of pre-eclampsia from 30 to 15% in the next pregnancy.

Further reading

Collins S, Arulkumaran S, et al. *Oxford Handbook of Obstetrics & Gynaecology.*
    3rd ed. Oxford: Oxford University Press; 2013.

MANAGEMENT OF LABOUR AND DELIVERY – QUESTIONS

SBAs

Question 1

With respect to the second stage of labour, which one of the following statements is true?

A. Cervical dilatation happens at 1 cm per hour.
B. Oxytocin should be used routinely in the second stage of labour in women with epidural.
C. A delayed second stage of labour is when the active second stage has lasted more than 2 hours in nulliparous and more than 1 hour in multiparous women.
D. Fetal heart should be auscultated at least every 15 minutes.
E. It ends with delivery of the fetal head.

Question 2

A 28-year-old G2 para 1 at 28 weeks' gestation attends the antenatal clinic to discuss vaginal birth after caesarean section (VBAC). She had a previous emergency caesarean section 3 years ago for undiagnosed breech in labour. Which one of the following is true concerning VBAC?

A. Intermittent monitoring during labour is recommended.
B. Risk of uterine rupture is 2%.
C. It is contraindicated in women with previous classical caesarean section.
D. The chances of successful vaginal birth is around 50%.
E. The risk of uterine rupture is 10 times higher if the labour is induced or augmented.

Question 3

With respect to fetal monitoring in labour, which one of the following statements is true?

A. Cardiotocography (CTG) is the recommended method of fetal monitoring in all labouring women.
B. Fetal blood sampling is indicated when the CTG is suspicious.
C. Normal baseline fetal heart at term is 110–160 bpm.
D. Absence of accelerations in an otherwise normal CTG is a non-reassuring feature.
E. Normal pH of fetus is 7.20.

Question 4

Reduced fetal movement is associated with the following risk factors except:

A. Fetal growth restriction
B. Placental insufficiency
C. Fetal neuromuscular conditions
D. Breech presentation
E. Small for gestational age

Question 5

With respect to the management of gestational hypertension in a G2 para 1 woman with a blood pressure of 145/96 mm Hg and no proteinuria at 35 weeks' gestation, which one of the following is the correct next step of management?

A. Admission to hospital
B. Weekly BP monitoring
C. Oral labetalol
D. Weekly blood tests
E. Induction of labour at 37 weeks' gestation

Question 6

A 35-year-old nulliparous woman at 36 weeks' gestation was diagnosed with pre-eclampsia. She complains of headaches and visual disturbances. Her blood pressure is 150/100 mmHg and Hb 10g/dl, platelets 90, ALT 88. She is at risk of the following complications except which one?

A. Cerebral haemorrhage
B. Placenta praevia
C. Pulmonary oedema
D. Eclampsia
E. Disseminated intravascular coagulation

Question 7

Which one of the following is true with regard to obstetric cholestasis?

A. Associated with long-term sequelae for mother and baby
B. Associated with stillbirth
C. Characterized by intense pruritus and skin rash
D. Associated abnormal liver function tests persist after birth
E. Typically presents in second trimester

Question 8

Which one of the following statements regarding analgesia in labour is true?

A. Intermittent auscultation of the fetal heart rate is acceptable for women using epidural analgesia.
B. Epidural analgesia can cause transient hypotension.
C. Oxytocin should be routinely used in the second stage of labour for women with epidural analgesia.
D. Epidural analgesia is less effective than opioids.
E. Epidural analgesia causes long-term backache.

Question 9

A 38-year-old woman presents to the maternity day assessment unit with a history of swollen feet, headache and blurring of vision at 30 weeks' gestation. Her BP is 160/100, pulse rate 88 bpm, oxygen saturation (SpO2) 99% on air and normal temperature. Uterine height measures 26 cm. Qualitative analysis of urine reveals 3 plusses of protein. What would be the diagnosis in this clinical context?

A. Migraine
B. Diabetic nephropathy
C. Glomerulonephritis
D. Unexplained proteinuria
E. Severe pre-eclampsia

Question 10

A 30-year-old woman presents to the labour ward with uterine contractions at 37 weeks' gestation. Her BP is 150/100 and quantitative analysis of urine shows 2 plusses of protein. Her bloods test results are otherwise normal. Which one of the statements below is false with regard to her management?

A. Hourly monitoring of BP
B. Intravenous access during labour and delivery
C. Start oral antihypertensive medication to stabilize BP
D. Epidural analgesia contraindicated
E. Oxytocin can be used for labour augmentation in cases of poor progress of labour

Question 11

Which of the following statements regarding bladder care is false?

A. Pregnant women should be encouraged to empty their bladder every 2–4 hours during labour to minimize the risk of retention of urine.
B. If the woman is unable to pass urine after 4 hours, an in-and-out catheter should be used to empty the bladder.
C. If repeat catheterization is required during labour, then one should consider inserting a Foley catheter.
D. If the woman has difficulties in emptying her bladder during or after labour, or requires a catheter, this is an indication for transfer from home to hospital for assessment.
E. Women should be taught self catheterization during pregnancy in anticipation of voiding difficulty in labour.

EMQs

OPTIONS FOR QUESTIONS 1–3

A. Passive second stage of labour
B. Latent first stage of labour
C. Delayed second stage of labour
D. Physiological third stage of labour
E. Active second stage of labour
F. Normal second stage of labour
G. Delayed third stage of labour
H. Established first stage of labour
I. Prolonged first stage of labour
J. Active third stage of labour

Instructions

For each clinical scenario below, choose the single most appropriate stage of labour from the above list of options. Each option may be used once, more than once or not at all.

1. A 30-year-old para 3 woman was admitted at term with regular uterine activity at 5 cm cervical dilatation and 4 hours later she delivered a female neonate with APGARs 9, 10, 10 at 1, 5 and 10 minutes. Syntometrine injection was given immediately after delivery and placenta with membranes was delivered completely 20 minutes after the delivery of the baby by continuous cord traction.
2. A 23-year-old para 3 woman was admitted after spontaneous rupture of membranes at 39 weeks' gestation. She is contracting 4 in 10 minutes and pushing involuntarily. On vaginal examination the cervix was fully dilated, vertex was 2 cm below the spines in direct occipito-anterior position with minimal caput and moulding.
3. A 30-year-old nulliparous woman was admitted at term with uterine contractions once in every 5 minutes. On examination, the fetus is in cephalic presentation with two fifths palpable per abdomen. The cervix is central, soft, fully effaced and 2 cm dilated with intact membranes.

OPTIONS FOR QUESTIONS 4–6

A. Augment with syntocinon
B. Administer prophylactic antibiotics
C. Allow vaginal delivery
D. Elective termination
E. HSV antibody testing
F. IV acyclovir
G. Instrumental delivery
H. No treatment at present
I. Oral acyclovir
J. Offer elective caesarean section
K. Perform caesarean section
L. Virology testing

Instructions

Each clinical scenario described below tests knowledge about the management of genital herpes. For each one select the single most appropriate management plan. Each option may be used once, more than once or not at all.

4. A 28-year-old woman presents to day assessment unit with primary active genital herpes simplex at 37 weeks' gestation.
5. A 29-year-old woman presents with spontaneous early labour at 38 weeks' gestation and has primary active genital herpes simplex infection.
6. A 29-year-old woman with history of recurrent genital herpes attends her antenatal appointment at 20 weeks. She is currently asymptomatic.

OPTIONS FOR QUESTIONS 7–9

A. Emergency caesarean section
B. Instrumental delivery
C. Augmentation of labour
D. Elective caesarean section
E. Oral augmentin
F. Induction of labour
G. Artificial rupture of membranes
H. Expectant management
I. Benzyl penicillin
J. Oral erythromycin

Instructions

For each clinical scenario below, choose the single most appropriate intervention from the above list of options. Each option may be used once, more than once or not at all.

7. A 32-year-old para 2 woman attends the labour ward in early labour at term with history of contractions once in every 5 minutes. On examination the head was five fifths palpable abdominally. On vaginal examination, the cervix was effaced, 4 cm dilated with bulging membranes, through which loops of cord could be felt.
8. A 30-year-old para 2 woman with dichorionic diamniotic twin pregnancy attends antenatal clinic at 36 weeks' gestation to discuss mode of delivery. Ultrasound that day confirmed that twin 1 was breech and twin 2 was in transverse position with normal growth, liquor and Dopplers of both babies.
9. A 30-year-old primigravida attends the maternity day assessment unit with history of spontaneous rupture of membranes (SROM) at 30 weeks' gestation. Speculum examination confirmed SROM. There is no uterine activity and the cardiotocography is normal. She was admitted for observation after the first dose of the dexamethasone injection.

OPTIONS FOR QUESTIONS 10–12

A. Await normal delivery
B. Elective caesarean section
C. Oxytocin augmentation
D. Immediate delivery by caesarean section
E. Induction of labour
F. Fetal blood sampling
G. Ventouse delivery
H. External cephalic version (ECV)
I. Breech delivery
J. Forceps delivery

Instructions

For each clinical scenario below, choose the single most appropriate intervention from the above list of options. Each option may be used once, more than once or not at all.

10. A 34-year-old primigravida with early onset pre-eclampsia presents with severe lower abdominal pain and a significant amount of ongoing fresh bleeding per vaginum at 34 weeks' gestation. Her pulse rate is 118 and BP is 100/60 mm Hg. On examination, the uterus is tender and tense with a pathological trace on cardiotocography (CTG).
11. A 26-year-old G2 para 1 woman at 37 weeks' gestation was referred by community midwife with a suspected breech presentation. She had a previous normal vaginal delivery and an uncomplicated antenatal period. Ultrasound confirmed extended breech presentation, normal amniotic fluid index and placenta is posterior high.
12. A 38-year-old G6 para 5 woman at term was brought in established labour at 8 cm cervical dilatation. Membranes rupture spontaneously with thick meconium stained liquor and, on vaginal examination, she is fully dilated with breech presentation. She has the urge to push and starts pushing involuntarily.

OPTIONS FOR QUESTIONS 13–15

A. Intermittent auscultation for 1 minute after contraction every 15 minutes
B. Intermittent auscultation for 1 minute after contraction every 10 minutes
C. Continuous CTG monitoring
D. No monitoring required
E. Intermittent auscultation for 1 minute after contraction every 5 minutes
F. Fetal scalp electrode monitoring
G. CTG monitoring for 20 minutes at admission
H. Fetal blood sampling
 I. CTG monitoring for 40 minutes at admission
 J. CTG monitoring every hour for 20 minutes

Instructions

For each of the scenarios below, choose the single most appropriate fetal monitoring method from the above list of options. Each option may be used once, more than once or not at all.

13. A 30-year-old para 2 woman with uncomplicated, low-risk pregnancy went into spontaneous labour at 39 weeks' gestation and was admitted at 4 cm cervical dilatation.
14. A 30-year-old para 2 woman with uncomplicated, low-risk pregnancy went into spontaneous labour at 39 weeks' gestation and was admitted at 4 cm cervical dilatation. The labour is progressing well and the fetal heart monitoring is being performed by intermittent auscultation. Spontaneous rupture of membranes reveals significant meconium stained liquor.
15. A 30-year-old para 2 woman with a BMI of 48 and no known medical problems went into spontaneous labour at 39 weeks' gestation was admitted at 5 cm cervical dilatation. She had spontaneous rupture of membranes an hour ago and CTG monitoring has been inadequate due to areas of loss of contact.

OPTIONS FOR QUESTIONS 16–18

A. Await normal delivery
B. Elective caesarean section
C. Augmentation with oxytocin
D. Immediate delivery by caesarean section
E. Induction of labour
F. Fetal blood sampling
G. Ventouse delivery
H. External cephalic version (ECV)
I. Amniotomy
J. Forceps delivery

Instructions

For each of the scenarios below, choose the single most appropriate action from the above list of options. Each option may be used once, more than once or not at all.

16. A 34-year-old nulliparous woman presents in established labour after spontaneous rupture of membranes and is contracting 3 in 10 minutes. She is 4 cm dilated and the fetal heart rate is normal. Four hours later she is still 4 cm dilated. The fetal heart is 140 beats per minute after a contraction.

17. A 33-year-old para 1 woman presents in spontaneous labour at 38 weeks' gestation and found to be 5 cm dilated with intact membranes. She is contracting 4 in 10 minutes and fetal heart monitoring is normal. On vaginal examination 4 hours later she was 6 cm dilated.

18. A 26-year-old para 1 woman presents in spontaneous labour at 39 weeks' gestation. She is 6 cm dilated, contracting 4 in 10 minutes and fetal heart is normal. Four hours later she is fully dilated and starts to push involuntarily with vertex 2 cm below the spines and good descent. The fetus is in occipito-anterior position and the fetal heart after a contraction is 140 beats per minute.

MCQs

1. With regard to caesarean section:
   A. If mother is HIV positive, a vaginal delivery is recommended rather than a caesarean section.
   B. If mother is HIV positive, a caesarean section is recommended when the viral load is zero.
   C. If the mother is HBsAg positive, a caesarean section is recommended rather than vaginal delivery.
   D. Caesarean section is recommended if the mother has cytomegalovirus infection.
   E. Caesarean section is recommended if the mother has syphilis.

2. Caesarean section possibly reduces the risk of:
   A. Respiratory morbidity in the newborn
   B. Perineal pain
   C. Uterovaginal prolapse
   D. Cerebral palsy
   E. Urinary incontinence

3. Regarding epidural analgesia in labour:
   A. It is associated with prolonged first stage.
   B. It is associated with prolonged second stage of labour.
   C. It is associated with long-term back problems.
   D. It is associated with fall in blood pressure following epidural top up.
   E. Woman can be mobile with epidural analgesia.

4. Continuous electronic fetal monitoring (EFM) is indicated during labour:
   A. If the pregnancy is low risk.
   B. If the woman opts to deliver at home.
   C. If the labour is being induced for small for dates.
   D. When syntocinon is used for augmentation of labour.
   E. When a woman is having vaginal birth after caesarean section (VBAC).

5. The following will cause abnormal fetal heart changes on CTG suggesting fetal distress during labour:
   A. Sitting position
   B. Hypotension secondary to epidural
   C. Scar dehiscence
   D. Cord compression
   E. Delivery in all fours position

6. Regarding pre-labour rupture of membranes (PROM):
   A. It promotes 90% women to go into spontaneous labour within 24 hours.
   B. It increases the risk of uterine infection.
   C. It can be diagnosed by performing a speculum examination.
   D. It increases the risk of pelvic infection.
   E. If prolonged, it increases the risk of maternal sepsis.

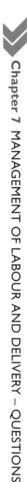

7. The following are indications for induction of labour:
   A. Post dates
   B. Prolonged rupture of membranes at term
   C. Placenta praevia
   D. Fetal growth restriction
   E. Previous 2 caesarean sections

8. The outcomes of IOL include:
   A. Vaginal delivery
   B. Failed IOL
   C. Uterine atony
   D. Uterine rupture
   E. Spontaneous rupture of membranes

9. The following measures should be taken to prevent transmission of HIV infection from mothers to their infants during pregnancy and labour:
   A. Decrease viral load by using anti-retroviral therapy and prophylaxis during pregnancy
   B. Fetal blood sampling is safe in such women
   C. Multiple cervical examinations is safe in such women
   D. Provide safer delivery practices
   E. Monitor and treat sexually transmitted infections

10. With regard to oxytocin:
    A. It is produced in the pituitary gland.
    B. Its action is antagonized by β agonist drugs.
    C. It can be used for induction of labour in women with rupture of membranes at term.
    D. It is used in the active management of third stage of labour to reduce postpartum blood loss.
    E. It is routinely used for all women in third stage of labour to reduce blood loss.

11. The diagnosis of pre-labour rupture of membranes (PROM) can be made by:
    A. History taking
    B. Speculum examination
    C. Ultrasound examination
    D. MRI scan
    E. CT scan

12. The following scenarios suggest that these women would require instrumental delivery during the second stage of labour:

A. A 29-year-old woman presents to the low risk maternity service with labour contractions at 39 weeks' gestation. She progresses to 10 cm cervical dilatation with cephalic presentation and fetal head is visible at the perineum. She has not started pushing yet but she indicates to the midwife that she can't push.

B. A 29-year-old woman presents to the labour ward at 41 weeks' gestation with regular uterine contractions. She gives a history of spontaneous rupture of membranes and her pad reveals thick meconium-stained liquor. Therefore, CTG was commenced for continuous fetal monitoring. She progresses well to full dilatation of the cervix and station of the fetal head is below spines. Thirty minutes later the midwife calls the oncall specialist registrar for review of CTG as it indicates pathological CTG. The registrar reviews the CTG and performs a fetal scalp blood sampling (FBS). The fetal scalp PH is <7.20.

C. A 29-year-old para 3 woman presents to labour ward at 42 weeks' gestation with regular uterine contractions and reduced fetal moments. Vaginal examination by midwife reveals high head and 3 cm cervical dilatation. The midwife asks the patient to mobilize and plans to reassess in 4 hours' time. The contractions get stronger and patient complains of sudden rupture of membranes and something coming out of the vagina. Examination by midwife reveals full dilatations of the cervix with station of the fetal head below spines. She also feels the umbilical cord below the fetal head.

D. A 29-year-old para 4 woman presents to the labour ward at 40 weeks' gestation with reduced fetal moment and regular uterine contractions. She also gives history of spontaneous rupture of membranes with thinly meconium stained liquor. As a consequence a CTG is commenced. The labour progresses very quickly to full dilatation with station of fetal head below spines. Review of CTG indicates suspicious CTG for more than 90 minutes.

E. A 29-year-old para 0 woman presents to the labour ward at 38 weeks' gestation with regular uterine contractions. She has an epidural sited for pain relief. The labour progresses well to full dilatation with fetal head at station +2. She pushes for an hour and the fetal head is visible at the perineum. A CTG was performed at this stage and is normal.

13. A 38-year-old para 1 woman attends the labour ward triage at 42 weeks' gestation with history of possible spontaneous rupture of membranes (SROM). She was considered low risk during her antenatal period. The following clinical management is appropriate in her case:

A. Thorough history taking is not important as she needs delivery anyway at 42 weeks' gestation

B. Perform a speculum examination to rule out SROM

C. Offer induction of labour if no signs of SROM on speculum examination

D. Offer induction of labour if signs of SROM on speculum examination

E. No need for induction of labour but await spontaneous onset of labour if no SROM

14. The following are correct NICE definitions for fetal heart rate changes:
    A. Bradycardia on CTG is defined as fetal heart beat >200 bpm for more than 3 minutes.
    B. Tachycardia on CTG is defined as fetal heart beat >160 bpm.
    C. Normal heart rate of the fetus is between 110 and 160.
    D. Typical variable decelerations on the CTG may indicate cord compression during labour.
    E. Occasional typical variable deceleration on CTG indicates fetal compromise.

15. A 29-year-old woman presents to the labour ward at 41 weeks' gestation with reduced fetal movements and regular uterine contractions. The labour progresses quickly to 8 cm cervical dilatation followed by spontaneous rupture of the membranes. The liquor at this stage is thick meconium stained and therefore a CTG is commenced for continuous fetal monitoring. One hour later, the midwife calls you to review the CTG as she feels it is pathological. The following management options would be reasonable in the case:
    A. Fetal blood scalp sampling as the CTG is pathological.
    B. Expedite delivery vaginally if the cervix is fully dilated and delivery is imminent.
    C. Expedite delivery if the fetal blood sampling shows pH of <7.20.
    D. Expedite delivery if the fetal blood sampling shows pH of >7.25.
    E. No need for any further action if the CTG continues to be pathological.

16. A 39-year-old woman has a spontaneous vaginal delivery at 36 weeks' gestation. The third stage of labour was managed actively. After 30 minutes the placenta remains undelivered and she has moderate vaginal bleeding. She was commenced on a 40-unit syntocinon infusion. Thirty minutes later the midwife informs the doctor that the placenta is still undelivered. Her management should include:
    A. Perform a full blood count and group and save
    B. Catheterize and keep the bladder empty
    C. Estimate the current blood loss and replace accordingly
    D. Inform anaesthetist that she will need hysterectomy
    E. Suction evacuation of the uterus

17. With regard to shoulder dystocia in labour:
    A. It can be easily prevented if the woman is assessed for risks factors during the antenatal period.
    B. Risk is increased if the woman is using epidural for analgesia.
    C. In 100% of cases, it occurs in babies who are macrosomic.
    D. Fetal complications such as brachial plexus palsy can occur during managing shoulder dystocia.
    E. Regular skills and drills are necessary to train midwifes and doctors to be prepared to handle such an emergency.

18. Regarding prelabour spontaneous rupture of membranes (SROM) at term:
    A. All women with SROM at term should be induced.
    B. Speculum examination should be performed to confirm SROM.
    C. Women should be informed that around 50–60% will go into spontaneous labour within 48 hours.
    D. Induction of labour should be offered after 24 hours of SROM if undelivered or does not go into labour spontaneously.
    E. Digital vaginal examination should be routinely performed to check cervical dilatation following SROM even in the absence of uterine contractions.

19. A 39-year-old woman presents to the labour ward at 39 weeks' gestation with regular uterine contractions. She has a BMI of 39 and a history of hypertension. She progresses to full dilatation in 20 hours and pushes for 90 minutes in second stage of labour. She requests assistance for delivery. A baby girl is born with the use of forceps and episiotomy. She used epidural for analgesia in labour. 6 hours later she could not pass urine. The following would be possible causes of urinary retention in her case:
    A. Psychological
    B. Urinary tract infection
    C. Operative delivery
    D. Hypertension
    E. Epidural use

20. A 29-year-old woman attends her antenatal appointment at 38 weeks' gestation. She is demanding elective caesarean section as her GP told her that vaginal delivery will cause vaginal prolapse in the future. The doctor in the antenatal clinic gives her the following advice regarding the ill effects of vaginal delivery on the perineum and pelvic floor:
    A. Most vaginal deliveries are associated with problems.
    B. Incontinence of flatus or faeces occurs in majority of women.
    C. Incontinence of flatus or faeces is usually associated with a combination of sphincter disruption and pudendal nerve trauma.
    D. Urogenital prolapse is usually due to routine use of episiotomy.
    E. The risk of genuine stress incontinence increases with increasing number of deliveries.

SBAs

Answer 1: C

The second stage of labour begins with full dilatation of the cervix and ends with the delivery of the baby. A delayed second stage is when the active second stage lasts ≥2 hours in nulliparous and ≥1 hour in multiparous women. Intermittent auscultation for fetal heart should happen at least every 5 minutes for at least a minute after a contraction. Routine use of oxytocin is not recommended in the second stage of labour.

Further reading

NICE clinical guideline 55. *Intrapartum care*. 2007. Available at: guidance.nice.org .uk/CG55

Answer 2: C

The success rate of a planned VBAC after one previous uncomplicated caesarean birth is 72–76%. The risk of uterine rupture is 50 per 10,000 VBAC and this risk increases two to three times higher if the labour is induced or augmented. VBAC should be conducted in a suitably staffed and equipped delivery suite, with continuous intrapartum monitoring and care with available resources for immediate caesarean section and neonatal resuscitation.

Further reading

RCOG Green-top guideline No. 45. *Birth after previous caesarean birth*. 2007. Available at: www.rcog.org.uk/womens-health/clinical-guidance /birth-after-previous-caesarean-birth-green-top-45

Answer 3: C

The recommended method of fetal monitoring in low-risk labouring women is intermittent auscultation of fetal heart and, in high-risk women, cardiotocography should be used. The normal baseline fetal heart rate is 110–160 bpm and the absence of accelerations in an otherwise normal CTG is of uncertain significance. FBS is indicated when the CTG is pathological and normal fetal pH is ≥7.25.

Further reading

Collins S, Arulkumaran S, et al. *Oxford Handbook of Obstetrics & Gynaecology*. 3rd ed. Oxford: Oxford University Press; 2013.

Answer 4: D

Fetal presentation has no effect on perception of fetal movements.

Further reading

RCOG Green-top guideline. *Reduced fetal movements*. 2011. Available at: www.rcog.org.uk/womens-health/clinical-guidance /reduced-fetal-movements-green-top-57

Answer 5: B

In women with mild gestational hypertension i.e. blood pressure between 140/90 to 149/99 mmHg, admission to hospital and antihypertensive treatment is not recommended. Blood pressure monitoring should not be more than once a week and proteinuria should be checked at each visit. Blood test monitoring except for the routine antenatal care is not recommended.

Further reading

NICE clinical guideline 107. *Hypertension in pregnancy*. 2011. Available at: www .nice.org.uk/nicemedia/live/13098/50418/50418.pdf

Answer 6: B

Placental abruption is a known complication, not placenta praevia.

Further reading

Collins S, Arulkumaran S, et al. *Oxford Handbook of Obstetrics & Gynaecology*. 3rd ed. Oxford: Oxford University Press; 2013.

Answer 7: B

Obstetric cholestasis, also known as intrahepatic cholestasis of pregnancy (IHCP), is a multifactorial condition of pregnancy characterized by intense pruritus in the absence of a skin rash, with abnormal liver function tests (LFTs), neither of which have an alternative cause and both of which remit following delivery. It typically presents after 30 weeks' gestation with itching of palms of the hand and soles of the feet, limbs and trunk. It is caused by intrahepatic cholestasis and has a recurrence rate of 45–90%. IHCP is associated with intrauterine fetal death, stillbirth and meconium passage. Delivery may be recommended at 37–38 weeks based on the severity of clinical or biochemical markers.

Further reading

RCOG Green-top guideline No. 43. *Obstetric cholestasis*. 2011. Available at: www.rcog.org.uk/files/rcog-corp/GTG43Obstetriccholestasis.pdf

Answer 8: B

Epidural analgesia is more effective than opioids and can cause transient hypotension but not long-term back problems. Routine oxytocin administration is not recommended during the second stage of labour for women with epidural analgesia but continuous electronic fetal monitoring is recommended.

Further reading

NICE clinical guideline 55. *Intrapartum care*. 2007. Available at: guidance.nice.org.uk/CG55

Answer 9: E

A pregnant woman presenting with raised blood pressure (BP 140/90 or more) with proteinuria with or without oedema after 20 weeks' gestation is defined as pre-eclampsia.

Facts about pre-eclampsia

- More common in a first pregnancy.
- The woman may give a past history of hypertension, renal disease, diabetes or family history.
- Women with a first-degree relative (mother or sister) who has a history of pre-eclampsia have a three-fold risk of developing pre-eclampsia.
- It is a common complication of pregnancy associated with significant fetal and maternal mortality and morbidity.
- An uncomplicated pregnancy with the same partner previously, confers a protective effect.
- A change of partner increases risk of pre-eclampsia.
- A change of partner after an affected pregnancy reduces risk.

Management principles of pre-eclampsia

- Management depends on the severity of the condition.
- Generally one should aim to prolong the pregnancy as long as possible.

- Severe pre-eclampisa – evidenced by symptoms, signs and abnormal blood tests – may need delivery after stabilization of the patient (control of blood pressure with anti-hypertensive drugs such as nifedipine, labetalol, hydralazine).
- Steroids should be considered in cases of premature delivery.
- Regular BP checks, FBC, U&Es, uric acid, LFTs, coagulation profile; 24-hour urine collection for protein; urine PCR for protein/creatinine ratio; fluid input and output charts should be kept
- Monitor the fetus-growth, Doppler scan and CTG.
- Delivery before 34 weeks' gestation may generally require delivery by caesarean section as the cervix would be unfavourable for vaginal delivery.
- At term, one should consider induction of labour unless the situation warrants urgent delivery because of maternal or fetal deterioration.
- Consider analgesia in labour and preferably epidural.
- Consider thromboprophylaxis after delivery and antiembolism stockings during labour.

Further reading

NICE clinical guideline 107. *Hypertension in pregnancy*. 2011. Available at: www .nice.org.uk/nicemedia/live/13098/50418/50418.pdf

Collins S, Arulkumaran S, et al. *Oxford Handbook of Obstetrics & Gynaecology*. 3rd ed. Oxford: Oxford University Press; 2013.

Answer 10: D

Monitoring and managing of women with PET during labour and puerperium

Mild or moderate HT or PET	Severe HT or PET	Antihypertensive medication	Analgesia	Intravenous fluids	Third stage of labour
Hourly BP	BP every 15 minutes	Continue oral medication in labour	PET is not a contra-indication to epidural providing platelets >80 × 10⁹/l.	IV access	Oxytocin should be given IM or IV 5 units
Continue antihypertensive oral medication	Stabilizing BP with oral treatment is important before considering delivery	If new onset of PET start with oral medication	If platelets <100 or liver function is abnormal clotting studies should be taken	Restrict intravenous fluids to 85 ml/hour	Avoid ergometrine if possible as there is risk of sudden exacerbation of HT

(Continued)

Mild or moderate HT or PET	Severe HT or PET	Antihypertensive medication	Analgesia	Intravenous fluids	Third stage of labour
Fetal monitoring with CTG	Fetal monitoring with CTG	If acute control necessary consider intravenous antihypertensives e.g. labetalol and hydrallazine	Epidural infusion provides better cardiovascular stability than epidural top-ups	Avoid overloading due to risk of pulmonary oedema and cardiac failure	Close monitoring of the blood pressure
Analgesia	Analgesia		Entonox and TENS machine can be used for analgesia		BP creeps up in a day or two again

Intramuscular (IM) or Intravenously (IV); Hypertension (HT)

All labour wards will have a protocol that should be followed.

Further reading

NICE clinical guideline 107. *Hypertension in pregnancy*. 2011. Available at: www .nice.org.uk/nicemedia/live/13098/50418/50418.pdf

Collins S, Arulkumaran S, et al. *Oxford Handbook of Obstetrics & Gynaecology*. 3rd ed. Oxford: Oxford University Press; 2013.

Answer 11: E

Bladder care during labour

- Women should be encouraged to void or empty their bladder at least every 4 hours during labour.
- Maximum time allowed without passing urine during labour should not exceed 6 hours.
- A full bladder during labour can affect delay in descent of the presenting part, inhibit uterine contraction, cause excessive pain, delay delivery of placenta and may predispose to postpartum haemorrhage by inhibition of uterine contractions.
- Women who require a forceps or ventouse for delivery, will need their bladder emptied prior to their delivery, so that trauma to the bladder is avoided.
- Women who had an epidural top-up or spinal anaesthesia are at increased risk of urinary retention and therefore an indwelling catheter should be kept in place for at least 12 hours post delivery.

Further reading

NICE clinical guideline No. 37. *Routine postnatal care of women and their babies*. 2006. Available at: www.nice.org.uk/nicemedia/pdf/CG37NICEguideline.pdf

EMQs

Answers 1–3

1. J

Active management of the third stage involves the routine use of uterotonic drugs, early clamping and cutting of the cord followed by controlled cord traction. Physiological management of third stage includes no routine use of uterotonic drugs, no clamping of the cord until pulsation has ceased and delivery of the placenta by maternal effort.

Further reading

NICE clinical guideline 55. *Intrapartum care: care of healthy women and their babies during childbirth.* 2007. Available at: www.nice.org.uk/nicemedia/pdf /IPCNICEGuidance.pdf

2. E

Active second stage of labour is when the baby is visible; or presence of expulsive contractions with a finding of full dilatation of the cervix or other signs of full dilatation of the cervix; or active maternal effort following confirmation of full dilatation of the cervix in the absence of expulsive contractions.

Further reading

NICE clinical guideline 55. *Intrapartum care: care of healthy women and their babies during childbirth.* 2007. Available at: www.nice.org.uk/nicemedia/pdf /IPCNICEGuidance.pdf

3. B

Latent first stage of labour is a period of time, not necessarily continuous, when there are painful contractions and there is some cervical change including cervical effacement and dilatation up to 4 cm. Established first stage of labour is when there are regular painful contractions and there is progressive cervical dilatation from 4 cm.

Further reading

NICE clinical guideline 55. *Intrapartum care: care of healthy women and their babies during childbirth.* 2007. Available at: www.nice.org.uk/nicemedia/pdf /IPCNICEGuidance.pdf

Answers 4–6

4. J

Women who have primary herpes simplex within 6 weeks of delivery are at an increased risk of transmitting the virus to fetus during vaginal delivery (30–60%) because of persistent viral shedding and lack of development of maternal antibodies to offer passive immunity to fetus. Therefore, elective caesarean section should be offered to these women at 39 weeks' gestation.

5. K

Women who present in labour with active primary herpes simplex are, again, at high risk of transmitting the virus to the fetus during delivery. Therefore, perform caesarean section to reduce the risk of transmission to the fetus.

If the primary infection occurs within 6 weeks of delivery or during labour, a caesarean section should be recommended. If vaginal delivery is opted for by a woman, artificial rupture of the membranes should be delayed or avoided, and intravenous acyclovir administered for mother during labour and neonate at birth.

6. H

The risk of transmission to the fetus is less (3%) with asymptomatic recurrent genital herpes. This patient is only at 20 weeks' gestation and, therefore, there is no need for any therapy at this point. If the same woman presents at term, she can be allowed to have vaginal delivery after discussion of the risks and benefits of transmission of the virus and also of vaginal delivery versus caesarean section. Due to lower risk of transmission of virus to the fetus with recurrent herpes, caesarean section is not routinely recommended. However, one should avoid fetal blood sampling and prolonged rupture of membranes. Caesarean section is only needed if genital lesions are present at delivery.

Further reading

RCOG Green-top guideline No. 30. *Management of genital herpes in pregnancy.* 2007. Available at: www.rcog.org.uk/womens-health/clinical-guidance /management-genital-herpes-pregnancy-green-top-30

Answers 7–9

7. A

The diagnosis is cord presentation and emergency caesarean section is recommended as the woman is in early labour and spontaneous rupture of membranes is likely to result in cord prolapse, an obstetric emergency.

Further reading

RCOG Green-top guideline No. 50. *Umbilical cord prolapse.* 2008. Available at: www .rcog.org.uk/files/rcog-corp/uploaded-files/GT50UmbilicalCordProlapse2008.pdf

Collins S, Arulkumaran S, et al. *Oxford Handbook of Obstetrics & Gynaecology.* 3rd ed. Oxford: Oxford University Press; 2013.

8. D

For uncomplicated dichorionic diamniotic twin pregnancies, delivery is recommended at 37–38 weeks' gestation. Normal vaginal delivery is recommended if the presenting twin is in cephalic presentation and caesarean section if the presenting twin is in non-vertex presentation.

Further reading

RCOG consensus views arising from the 50th study group. *Multiple pregnancy.* Available at: www.rcog.org.uk/files/rcog-corp/uploaded-files /StudyGroupConsensusViewsMultiplePregnancy.pdf

Collins S, Arulkumaran S, et al. *Oxford Handbook of Obstetrics & Gynaecology.* 3rd ed. Oxford: Oxford University Press; 2013.

9. J

In women with preterm prelabour rupture of membranes expectant management is the mainstay of treatment if there are no signs of infection and the woman is not in labour. Antenatal corticosteroids should be administered and prophylactic erythromycin should be given for 10 days following the diagnosis of PPROM to minimize the risk of chorioamnionitis, neonatal infection and to prolong the pregnancy.

Further reading

RCOG Green-top guideline No 44. *Preterm prelabour rupture of membranes.* 2010. Available at: www.rcog.org.uk/files/rcog-corp/GTG44PPROM28022011.pdf

Collins S, Arulkumaran S, et al. *Oxford Handbook of Obstetrics & Gynaecology.* 3rd ed. Oxford: Oxford University Press; 2013.

Answers 10–12

10. D

The likely diagnosis is antepartum haemorrhage secondary due to placental abruption with active ongoing bleeding and signs of maternal and fetal compromise. Hence, immediate delivery by caesarean section is indicated unless the cervix is fully dilated and delivery can be achieved vaginally.

Further reading

Collins S, Arulkumaran S, et al. *Oxford Handbook of Obstetrics & Gynaecology.* 3rd ed. Oxford: Oxford University Press; 2013.

11. H

Women should be counselled that ECV reduces the chance of breech presentation at delivery and thereby reduces their chances of having a caesarean section. External cephalic version should be offered to women with breech presentation to minimize the risk of caesarean section.

Further reading

RCOG Green-top guideline No. 20a. *External cephalic version and reducing the incidence of breech presentation.* 2010. Available at: www.rcog.org.uk/files /rcog-corp/uploaded-files/GT20aExternalCephalicVersion.pdf

RCOG Green-top guideline No. 20b. *The management of breech presentation.* 2006. Available at: www.rcog.org.uk/files/rcog-corp/GtG%20no%2020b%20 Breech%20presentation.pdf

12. I

It is prudent to prepare for the breech vaginal delivery as she is likely to deliver shortly after the situation has been explained to her. A practitioner skilled in the conduct of labour with breech presentation and vaginal breech birth should be present at all vaginal breech births.

Further reading

RCOG Green-top guideline No. 20b. *The management of breech presentation.* 2006. Available at: www.rcog.org.uk/files/rcog-corp/GtG%20no%2020b%20 Breech%20presentation.pdf

Answers 13–15

13. A

During established first stage of labour, intermittent auscultation of the fetal heart after a contraction for a minimum of one minute should take place at least every 15 minutes.

Further reading

NICE clinical guideline 55. *Intrapartum care: care of healthy women and their babies during childbirth.* 2007. Available at: www.nice.org.uk/nicemedia/pdf /IPCNICEGuidance.pdf

14. C

Continuous electronic fetal monitoring should be advised for women with significant meconium stained liquor, which is either dark green or black, thick, tenacious containing lumps of meconium.

Further reading

NICE clinical guideline 55. *Intrapartum care: care of healthy women and their babies during childbirth.* 2007. Available at: www.nice.org.uk/nicemedia/pdf /IPCNICEGuidance.pdf

15. F

Women with a BMI >35 become high risk and should have continuous electronic fetal monitoring in labour. If there are no contraindications, and continuous monitoring is not feasible due to loss of contact with external monitors, fetal scalp electrode monitoring is the method of choice.

Further reading

NICE clinical guideline 55. *Intrapartum care: care of healthy women and their babies during childbirth.* 2007. Available at: www.nice.org.uk/nicemedia /pdf/IPCNICEGuidance.pdf

Answers 16–18

16. C

When there is a delay in the established first stage of labour, the use of oxytocin should be considered and advice should be sought from an obstetrician. Women should be informed that oxytocin use after spontaneous rupture of membranes will bring forward her time of birth, but will not influence the mode of delivery or other outcomes.

Further reading

NICE clinical guideline 55. *Intrapartum care: care of healthy women and their babies during childbirth.* 2007. Available at: www.nice.org.uk/nicemedia/pdf /IPCNICEGuidance.pdf

17. I

There is a delay in the established first stage of labour where there is only 1 cm dilatation in 4 hours in a parous woman. As per NICE intrapartum care guidance, amniotomy (ARM) should be considered for all women with intact membranes following an explanation of the procedure and advice that it will shorten her labour by about an hour, as well as increasing the strength and pain of her contractions.

Further reading

NICE clinical guideline 55. *Intrapartum care: care of healthy women and their babies during childbirth.* 2007. Available at: www.nice.org.uk/nicemedia/pdf /IPCNICEGuidance.pdf

18. A

There is a good progress of labour during the established first stage of labour and during the second stage with no evidence of fetal compromise, hence no intervention is necessary and one should await the vaginal delivery to take place.

Further reading

NICE clinical guideline 55. *Intrapartum care: care of healthy women and their babies during childbirth.* 2007. Available at: www.nice.org.uk /nicemedia/pdf/IPCNICEGuidance.pdf

MCQs

1A: False
1B: False – Vaginal delivery is considered when the viral load is zero or <50 copies.
1C: False
1D: False
1E: False

Many women with HIV infection will have caesarean section because it reduces the risk of vertical transmission, but not for those with hepatitis B or C.

Further reading

RCOG Green-top guideline No. 39. *HIV in pregnancy, management.* 2010. Available at: www.rcog.org.uk/womens-health/clinical-guidance /management-hiv-pregnancy-green-top-39

NICE clinical guidance 13. *Caesarean section.* 2004. Available at: www.nice.org.uk /nicemedia/pdf/CG013NICEguideline.pdf

2A: False
2B: True
2C: True
2D: False – Caesarean section has not reduced the rate of cerebral palsy in children when compared with vaginal delivery.
2E: True

Further reading

RCOG Green-top guideline No. 45. *Birth after previous caesarean birth.* 2007. Available at: www.rcog.org.uk/womens-health/clinical-guidance /birth-after-previous-caesarean-birth-green-top-45

NICE clinical guidance 13. *Caesarean section.* 2004. Available at: www.nice.org.uk /nicemedia/pdf/CG013NICEguideline.pdf

3A: False
3B: True
3C: False
3D: True
3E: True

Epidural analgesia

- It does not increase the length of first stage of labour.
- It does not increase the chance of caesarean delivery.
- It is not associated with long-term back pain problems.
- It increases the chance of an operative vaginal delivery.
- Electronic fetal monitoring should be undertaken for 30 minutes at the initiation of the epidural and after each additional bolus.

- Most units have protocols to monitor the fetus continuously once the epidural is sited.
- Walking is possible with mobile epidurals.
- Drop-in blood pressure is seen following epidural top-up and can also be associated with CTG abnormality.

Further reading

NICE clinical guideline 55. *Intrapartum care.* 2007. Available at: guidance.nice.org
.uk/CG55

4A: False
4B: False
4C: True
4D: True
4E: True

Monitoring of the fetal heart rate (FHR) in labour aims to identify hypoxia before it is sufficient to lead to long-term poor neurological outcomes for babies.

Pregnant women can be divided into:

a. High risk for pregnancy and high risk for labour
b. Low risk for pregnancy and high risk for labour
c. Low risk for pregnancy and low risk for labour

The first two categories require continuous CTG or electronic fetal monitoring (EFM). The last category requires intermittent auscultation unless the clinical situation changes during labour. Performing a CTG for low-risk women in labour has not shown any improvement in fetal outcome.

It is important to explain the risks and benefits to women who require continuous intrapartum fetal monitoring.

Indications for continuous electronic fetal monitoring (EFM) in labour

- Women who are high risk for pregnancy and high risk for labour
  - Pregnancy-induced hypertension and pre-eclampsia
  - Diabetes
  - Any other medical disorder
  - High-risk fetus – prematurity, intra-uterine growth retardation (IUGR), oligohydramnios, abnormal ultrasound scan/Dopplers.
  - Any high-risk pregnancy
  - Previous caesarean section
  - Multiple pregnancy
  - Recurrent ante-partum haemorrhage
  - Significant ante-partum haemorrhage
  - Breech presentation
  - Women requiring syntocinon

- Meconium-stained liquor
- Substance abuse e.g. cocaine, cannabis and heavy smokers
- Women induced for reduced fetal movements and clinically small for dates

- Women who are low risk for pregnancy but high risk for labour
  - Meconium-stained liquor
  - Prolonged SROM
  - Use of syntocinon for augmentation of labour
  - During and following epidural analgesia
  - Vaginal bleeding during labour with suspicion of antepartum haemorrhage
  - Abnormal FHR detected by intermittent auscultation (less than 110 bpm; greater than 160 bpm; any deceleration heard after a contraction)
  - Maternal pyrexia (38.0°C once or 37.5°C on two occasions, 2 hours apart)
  - Women induced for reduced fetal movements and clinically small for dates
- Maternal request

Further reading

NICE clinical guideline 55. *Intrapartum care*. 2007. Available at: guidance.nice.org .uk/CG55

5A: False
5B: True
5C: True – If there is a suspicion of scar dehiscence, the woman would need urgent caesarean section as it is dangerous to both mother and the fetus (can lead to fetal death).
5D: True – Change of position may help sometimes, unless it is due to severe oligohydramnious, anhydramnious or cord prolapse.
5E: False
CTG abnormalities during labour are not uncommon. One should treat the possible cause if it is known.

- If the cause is dehydration
  - Check urine ketones and treat dehydration if suspected
- If cause is hypotension secondary to epidural
  - Check BP post epidural and give 500ml of crystalloid if appropriate
- If the cause is maternal pyrexia and tachycardia
  - Consider infection screen including FBC, CRP and blood cultures
  - Start intravenous antibiotics as per unit protocol
  - Administer 1 gm intravenous paracetomol every 8 hours
  - Ensure adequate hydration
  - Consider delivery if fetal compromise is suspected
- If the cause is aorta-caval compression
  - Maternal position should be changed to left lateral to avoid aorta-caval compression if maternal hypotension evident
- If the cause is cord compression
  - Change position to left or right lateral
- If the cause is uterine hyperstimulation

- Consider tocolysis with 0.25 mg terbutaline subcutaneously
- Terbutaline can be repeated after 15 minutes if necessary
- Obtain informed consent and document in the notes
- If this occurs following injudicious use of syntocinon, syntocinon should be reduced or stopped depending on the number of contractions and titrated to achieve not more than four or five contractions in 10 minutes

Document the management plan and the CTG should be reviewed again in 30–40 minutes by the doctor.

Further reading

NICE clinical guideline 55. *Intrapartum care*. 2007. Available at: guidance.nice.org. uk/CG55

6A: False – 60% would go into spontaneous labour within 24 hours.
6B: True
6C: True – A speculum examination should be performed to confirm the PROM unless it is obvious. A digital vaginal exam should be avoided in the absence of contractions to minimize the risk of infection (chorioamnionitis).
6D: True
6E: True – One has to be vigilant about the signs of maternal sepsis in women with prolonged rupture of membranes. Maternal sepsis is the leading cause of maternal death according to the last CEMACE report (2006–2008) in the UK.
Most women (60%) with PROM would go into spontaneous labour within 24 hours. Therefore, women can be managed expectantly for the initial 24 hours. However, she should be warned about the signs of infection and advised to take temperature every 4 hourly. If she feels unwell and has raised temperature or reduced fetal movements she should seek immediate medical advice.

If she does not go into labour within 24 hours, induction of labour is recommended due to increased risk of infection to both the fetus (the risk of serious neonatal infection is about 1%) and the mother. Women with prolonged rupture of the membranes (24–36 hours) may need prophylactic antibiotics during labour until delivery, even if there is no clinical evidence of infection. Benzyl penicillin is used for prophylaxis. In a woman who is allergic to penicillin, clindamycin is recommended. The criteria for antibiotic use may differ in different maternity units.

Further reading

NICE clinical guideline 55. *Intrapartum care*. 2007. Available at: guidance.nice.org. uk/CG55

7A: True
7B: True
7C: False
7D: True
7E: False

One in five deliveries in the UK is induced. Induction of labour (IOL) will be offered for women who go past 41 weeks' gestation. It is commonly undertaken when labour fails to start spontaneously by 10 days past the due date. If the woman chooses not to be induced at this stage then from 42 weeks they should be offered:

- twice-weekly checks of their baby's heartbeat (CTG) using the electronic fetal heart rate monitor;
- a single ultrasound scan to check the depth of amniotic fluid (or water's) surrounding their baby; and
- umbilical artery Doppler to check the end-diastolic flow.

An ultrasound scan in early pregnancy (before 20 weeks) can help to determine the due date more accurately and reduces the chances of unnecessary induction.

The other indications for IOL include:

- Maternal indications
  - Preterm prelabour rupture of membranes
  - Prelabour rupture of membranes at term
  - Pre-eclampsia
  - Diabetes in pregnancy
  - Other medical conditions in pregnancy
  - Are >40 years: induce at term (40 weeks)
- Fetal indications
  - Fetal growth restriction
- Intrauterine fetal death

Methods of IOL

There are a variety of methods that can be used to induce labour. In the community or NHS hospital setting a membrane sweep can be performed. It has been shown to increase the chances of labour starting spontaneously within the next 48 hours and can reduce the need for other methods of induction of labour. This method is not recommended if the membranes have ruptured already.

In the hospital, IOL can be started in two ways:

1. Prostaglandins (PGE2) vaginally (tablet or pessary or gel). This helps the cervix to soften, dilate, and initiate the onset of labour.
2. Artificial rupture of membranes (ARM). This is usually followed by a syntocinon augmentation of labour.

The fetal heart is monitored (CTG) before initiation of IOL with prostaglandins. After the first dose of prostaglandin the cervix is usually examined after 6 hours to perform an ARM. If this is not possible a second dose of prostaglandins can be offered to the patient unless there are no concerns with the fetal wellbeing on CTG.

There is no evidence to suggest that labour induced with prostaglandins is any more painful than labour that has started spontaneously. However, prostaglandins can cause vaginal soreness.

Further reading

NICE clinical guideline 70. *Induction of labour*. 2008. Available at: publications.nice.
org.uk/induction-of-labour-cg70

8A: True – The outcome of IOL can be vaginal delivery, instrumental delivery,
caesarean section or failed IOL.

8B: True – Failed IOL can occur in 15% of women with an unfavourable
cervical examination.

8C: False – IOL can cause uterine hyperstimulation (>5 contractions in
10 minutes). This is seen in 1–5% of women who undergo IOL. Often this requires
no intervention but treatment is indicated if it leads to fetal distress, which is
usually seen while monitoring the fetus with CTG. Terbutaline 0.25 mg (tocolytic
agent) is given subcutaneously to reduce the contractions.

8D: True – A rare obstetric emergency which requires immediate caesarean section.

8E: False – The aim of IOL is to get women into labour. The first step is rupture of
membranes, which is generally artificial rupture of membranes. However, some
women may already have spontaneous rupture of membranes (SROM) and would
need augmentation. One should be careful while performing ARM as there is
a small risk of umbilical cord prolapse through the cervix. This is an obstetric
emergency and the delivery of the baby should be performed immediately.

Further reading

NICE clinical guideline 70. *Induction of labour*. 2008. Available at: publications.nice
.org.uk/induction-of-labour-cg70

NICE clinical guideline 55. *Intrapartum care*. 2007. Available at: guidance.nice.org
.uk/CG55

9A: True
9B: False
9C: False – Cervical examinations should be kept to a minimum.
9D: True
9E: True

Antenatal measures to reduce the risk of HIV transmission from mother to fetus

- Counselling for HIV
- Anti-retroviral therapy to treat maternal HIV and reduce the viral load
- Diagnose and treat sexually transmitted infections
- Promote safer sex practices
- Provide infant-feeding counselling and support

Safe delivery practices to reduce the risk of HIV transmission from mother to infant

- Avoid routine rupture of membranes
- Avoid prolonged labour

- Minimize cervical examinations
- Minimize exposure of fetus to maternal blood and body fluids
- Avoid invasive monitoring e.g. fetal blood sampling, fetal scalp electrode and STAN monitoring
- Avoid unnecessary trauma during childbirth e.g. difficult forceps or ventouse delivery
- Avoid unresolved sexually transmitted infections
- Administer antiretroviral prophylaxis during labour
- Perform elective caesarean section when safe and feasible
- Perform emergency caesarean section early at the onset of labour or membrane rupture
- Vaginal delivery can be considered if the viral load is zero or less than 50 copies
- Use safe transfusion practices

Post partum measures to reduce the risk of transmission to fetus

- Avoid breastfeeding
- Replacement feeding
- Encourage anti-retroviral prophylaxis for infant if indicated

Further reading

RCOG Green-top guideline No. 39. *Management of HIV in pregnancy*. 2010. Available at: www.rcog.org.uk/womens-health/clinical-guidance /management-hiv-pregnancy-green-top-39

Collins S, Arulkumaran S, et al. *Oxford Handbook of Obstetrics & Gynaecology*. 3rd ed. Oxford: Oxford University Press; 2013.

10A: False
10B: True
10C: True
10D: True
10E: False

Oxytocin (synthetic version is called syntocinon) is produced by the supra-optic and paraventricular nuclei and is transported to the posterior pituitary gland via neuronal axons to be stored and released by the pituitary gland. It can be used for induction of labour in women with spontaneous rupture of membranes, augmentation of labour in women with poor progress of labour and active management of third stage of labour to prevent postpartum haemorrhage. It need not be used for women who opt for physiological third stage of labour. During spontaneous and augmented labour it promotes prostaglandin (PGF2α) release from the decidua and enhances uterine contractions and cervical ripening. β agonists promote uterine relaxation and are therefore used in women presenting with a preterm labour to counteract uterine activity. The indications for β agonist usage include: (a) allowing time while administering steroids to mother to promote fetal lung maturity; or (b) if the fetus requires intrauterine transfer to another hospital.

One should be cautious if a labour is augmented and there is poor progress. Further use of oxytocin may not be effective as prolonged administration of oxytocin down-regulates its own receptor. Prolonged use of oxytocin also causes vasodilatation, hypotension, tachycardia and hyponatraemia. Therefore, one should be cautious while administering repeated intravenous (IV) boluses of oxytocin in a woman with massive postpartum haemorrhage (PPH). This can cause sudden collapse in an already compromised woman and may lead to death. On the other hand it can also cause water retention due to some of its antidiuretic action.

As explained earlier oxytocics like syntocinon are uterotonics. They promote contraction of the uterine muscle and therefore reduce postpartum blood loss. The most common drugs used in the active management of third stage of labour include an intravenous (IV) bolus of oxytocin or an intramuscular (IM) injection of syntometrine (combination of oxytocin + ergometrine preparation). The other uses of oxytocin include management of excessive bleeding after miscarriage or abortion. The side effects of oxytocin include nausea, vomiting, cramping, light-headedness, water retention and hyponatraemia.

Further reading

NICE clinical guideline 55. *Intrapartum care*. 2007. Available at: guidance.nice.org.uk/CG55

Collins S, Arulkumaran S, et al. *Oxford Handbook of Obstetrics & Gynaecology*. 3rd ed. Oxford: Oxford University Press; 2013.

11A: False – Diagnosis is suspected on the basis of history and confirmed by speculum examination.
11B: True – Sterile speculum examination is the gold standard for confirmation or exclusion of rupture of membranes. It allows assessment of liquor colour and helps to rule out cord prolapse or presentation. Where there is a persuasive history of rupture of membranes but no liquor seen even on coughing, then a speculum examination can be repeated after 1 hour of the patient lying supine, which allows liquor to pool in the vagina.
11C: False – Ultrasound measurement of the amniotic fluid volume can neither confirm nor exclude rupture of membranes; it can simply assess the current amniotic fluid volume.
11D: False
11E: False

Further reading

Collins S, Arulkumaran S, et al. *Oxford Handbook of Obstetrics & Gynaecology*. 3rd ed. Oxford: Oxford University Press; 2013.

12A: False
12B: True
12C: True
12D: True
12E: False

Indications for operative vaginal delivery can be divided into maternal and fetal causes.

- Maternal causes
  - Maternal exhaustion due to labour or maternal distress
  - Limit time in second stage of labour due to medical conditions including moderate-to-severe cardiac disease, cerebrovascular malformations and hypertensive crisis
  - Lack of maternal effort to push due to medical conditions including myasthenia gravis, and spinal cord injury (paraplegia and quadriplegia)
  - Inability to push because of lack of consciousness
- Fetal causes
  - Presumed fetal distress or compromise
  - Bradycardia or fetal heart beat <100 beats per minute for more than 3 minutes
- Fetal scalp blood sampling with pH <7.20 indicates severe fetal distress. In this situation delivery should be expedited (within 30 minutes of diagnosis and decision). One should also take caution not to perform a difficult instrumental delivery because of the increased risk of intracranial bleeding.

A paediatrician should be present at delivery. After delivery, paired cord blood sampling for pH and base excess should be collected.

Inadequate progress in second stage of labour

- Nulliparous women: lack of continuing progress for 3 hours (total of active and passive stage) of second stage with regional anaesthesia or 2 hours without regional anaesthesia
- Multiparous women: lack of continuing progress for 2 hours (total of active and passive stage) of second stage with regional anaesthesia or 1 hour without regional anaesthesia

Further reading

RCOG Green-top guideline No. 26. *Operative vaginal delivery*. 2011. Available at: www.rcog.org.uk/womens-health/clinical-guidance/operative-vaginal-delivery-green-top-26

RCOG consent advice No. 11. *Operative vaginal delivery*. 2010. Available at: www.rcog.org.uk/operative-vaginal-delivery-consent-advice-11

NICE clinical guideline 55. *Intrapartum care*. 2007. pp 47–50. Available at: guidance.nice.org.uk/CG55

13A: False
13B: True
13C: True
13D: True
13E: False – She is already 42 weeks' gestation and therefore needs induction of labour even if there is no SROM. The risk of intrauterine death, meconium stained liquor and oligohydramnios increases with postmaturity.

Fetal and maternal risks increase after 41 weeks' gestation (prolonged pregnancy). Fetal risk includes increased perinatal mortality (PNM) rate and morbidity, increased stillbirth rate, meconium aspiration and shoulder dystocia. Maternal risks include increase in operative delivery. Therefore, NICE recommends routine induction of labour after 41 weeks' gestation as evidence suggests it would decrease perinatal (PNM) mortality and morbidity as well as decrease instrumental and caesarean delivery rate. If the woman declines induction of labour, monitoring should be offered in the form of daily fetal kick count, daily CTG and weekly amniotic fluid measurements. However, women should be thoroughly counselled that the commonly used tests for fetal wellbeing – including fetal kick count, CTG, amniotic fluid measurements, umbilical artery Doppler – do not reliably predict compromise in this situation.

Further reading

NICE clinical guideline 70. *Induction of labour*. 2008. Available at: publications.nice. org.uk/induction-of-labour-cg70

14A: False – Bradycardia is defined as fetal heart beat below 100 bpm, lasting for >3 minutes.

14B: True
14C: True
14D: True
14E: False

The four normal features of CTG trace:

1. Baseline: fetal heart rate between 110–160 bpm
2. Variability: should be >5 bpm
3. Acceleration: should be present (defined as increase of the fetal heart beat of more than 15 beats above baseline and lasting for 15 seconds)
4. Decelerations: should be absent (defined as decrease in the fetal heart beat of more than 15 beats below baseline and lasting for 15 seconds)

NICE definitions of normal, suspicious and pathological FHR traces

- Normal: an FHR trace in which all four features are classified as reassuring.
- Suspicious: an FHR trace with one feature classified as non-reassuring and the remaining features classified as reassuring. In this situation, one can observe for some time (40 minutes) but there should be a clear plan if the CTG continues to be suspicious.
- Pathological: an FHR trace with two or more features classified as non-reassuring or one or more classified as abnormal. This kind of CTG trace indicates presumed fetal distress or compromise. Therefore, one should either deliver the fetus within 30 minutes if indicated or perform fetal blood sampling to check if the fetus is compromised. This is a clinical decision and would depend on the overall clinical circumstances.

Further reading

NICE clinical guideline 55. *Intrapartum care*. 2007. pp 47–50. Available at: guidance
.nice.org.uk/CG55

15A: True
15B: True
15C: True
15D: False
15E: False

NICE recommends fetal blood sampling when the CTG is pathological
(contraindications include bradycardia due to cord prolapse, uterine rupture,
abruptio placenta and in certain maternal infection such as hepatitis B and HIV).
NICE recommends that the results of FBS should be interpreted carefully taking
into account of previous pH measurement, the rate of progress in labour and the
clinical features of the woman and baby.

Interpretation of fetal blood sample result (pH)

- ≥ 7.25: normal FBS result
- 7.21–7.24: borderline FBS result (may require repeating in 30–60 minutes)
- ≤ 7.20: abnormal FBS result (needs urgent delivery)

Fetal blood sampling should be performed when fetal compromise is suspected
(which is interpreted on CTG as pathological).

- After a normal FBS result, sampling should be repeated no more than one hour later
  if the FHR trace remains pathological or sooner if there are further abnormalities.
- After a borderline FBS result, sampling should be repeated no more than
  30 minutes later if the FHR trace remains pathological or sooner if there are
  further abnormalities. The time taken to take a fetal blood sample needs to be
  considered when planning repeat samples.
- If the FHR trace remains unchanged and the FBS result is stable after
  the second test, a third/further sample may be deferred unless additional
  abnormalities develop on the trace.
- Where a third FBS is considered necessary, a consultant obstetric opinion
  should be sought.

Further reading

NICE clinical guideline 55. *Intrapartum care*. 2007. pp 47–50. Available at: guidance.
nice.org.uk/CG55

16A: True
16B: True
16C: True
16D: False
16E: False

The placenta is considered to be retained if undelivered 30 minutes following vaginal delivery. One should ensure that the woman has a large bore cannula and group and save if she is bleeding vaginally. If she is bleeding excessively, a cross-match for 2–4 units of packed cell volume (PCV) should be requested. Her bladder should be emptied to ensure proper uterine contractions. She should be kept nil by mouth in case she needs manual removal of placenta (MROP) under general anaesthesia.

If the bleeding is mild and the woman is clinically stable, the following options can be tried:

- Further controlled cord traction (CCT) can be tried to check if the placenta can be delivered (often the placenta can be trapped in the cervix or just above the cervix following cervical contraction).
- Oxytocin infusion (20 units in 20ml of normal saline) through umbilical cord (umbilical vein).
- The woman should be encouraged to breastfeed to promote uterine contraction so that placenta is separated and expelled and bleeding is reduced (breastfeeding promotes release of the oxytocin from the pituitary gland and therefore promotes uterine contraction).

If the bleeding is active, MROP should be performed under general anaesthesia. Informed consent should be taken before the procedure and the cavity should be checked to ensure it is empty after the procedure. She would also need prophylactic intravenous antibiotics at the time of induction to decrease the risk of uterine infection. After the procedure, the uterus should be kept contracted by using syntocinon 40 units infusion as well as by insertion of rectal misoprostol (600–1000 μg).

Further reading

NICE clinical guideline 55. *Intrapartum care.* 2007. Available at: guidance.nice.org.uk/CG55

Collins S, Arulkumaran S, et al. *Oxford Handbook of Obstetrics & Gynaecology.* 3rd ed. Oxford: Oxford University Press; 2013.

17A: False – Shoulder dystocia can be anticipated or predicted if the woman is assessed for risk factors during the antenatal period. It is not preventable but can be anticipated in women with fetal macrosomia. The other risk factors for shoulder dystocia include maternal obesity, diabetes (increases the risk of shoulder dystocia by more than 70%), fetal macrosomia, previous shoulder dystocia (12% recurrence in future pregnancies), prolonged labour (labour progresses normally in 70% of women) and difficult instrumental delivery.
17B: False – It is not related to the use of analgesia.
17C: False – 50% of shoulder dystocia occurs in babies with normal birth weight.
17D: True – Fetal complications include birth trauma, brachial plexus injury (due to excessive neck traction), fracture clavicle or humerus while the maternal complications include genital tract trauma and postpartum haemorrhage.

17E: True – It is a requirement for all NHS trusts that doctors and midwifes should undergo skills and drills on a yearly basis to be able to be prepared to handle various obstetric emergencies including shoulder dystocia. It is also a Clinical Negligence Scheme for Trusts (CNST) requirement.

Shoulder dystocia is defined as failure to deliver the shoulders after the head has been delivered. The incidence is 0.5–2% of all vaginal deliveries.

Early induction of labour in women with fetal macrosomia does not reduce either shoulder dystocia or the caesarean section rate. Elective caesarean section is not recommended for women with fetal macrosomia on scan as this has not been shown to decrease operative delivery or shoulder dystocia or birth trauma. However, this rule does not apply to diabetic women. It is reasonable to do a planned caesarean section in diabetic women with birth weight more than 4500 gm.

Further reading

RCOG Green-top guideline No. 42. *Shoulder dystocia.* 2005. Available at: www.rcog .org.uk/womens-health/clinical-guidance/shoulder-dystocia-green-top-42

The American College of Obstetricians and Gynaecologists. *Shoulder dystocia.* 2013. Available at: www.acog.org/Resources_And_Publications

18A: False
18B: True
18C: True
18D: True
18E: False

Diagnosis and investigation of prelabour spontaneous rupture of membranes (SROM) term

- Take a thorough history of SROM including colour, odour and duration.
- Confirm SROM by doing a speculum examination. One can also exclude a cord prolapse.
- Digital examination is not recommended in view of introducing infection, unless the woman is in labour.
- Full blood count and CRP are not routinely indicated unless the woman gives history of prolonged SROM.
- Take a high vaginal swab (HVS).
- Check presentation and fetal wellbeing.

Counselling and management of women with SROM at term

- Counsel women regarding risk including 1% serious risk of neonatal infection and chorioamnionitis if prolonged SROM.
- Pros and cons of expectant management versus immediate induction of labour should be discussed with women and an informed choice made by patient.
- Expectant management for 24 hours after SROM is reasonable in the absence of infection or fetal compromise and around 60% will go into labour within 24 hours of SROM.

- Induction of labour should be offered 24 hours after SROM.
- Women should be advised to take their temperature 4 hourly at home.
- Bathing and showering are not associated with an increase in infection.
- Sexual intercourse may be associated with an increase in infection.
- The woman should report any reduced fetal movements.
- Antibiotics are not routinely advised in the absence of infection while they are definitely indicated in the presence of infection even before 24 hours.

Further reading

NICE clinical guideline 55. *Intrapartum care*. 2007. Available at: guidance.nice.org .uk/CG55

19A: False
19B: True
19C: True
19D: False
19E: True

Possible causes of urinary retention in labour or following delivery can be related to the pregnancy itself; to the labour (prolonged labour); to the mode of delivery (operative vaginal delivery, which includes use of forceps or ventouse for delivery); to the type of analgesia used (epidural can predispose to urinary retention); to any possible neurological damage (prolonged labour and pushing can cause devascularization of the bladder neck and nerve damage); to any pre-existing conditions including diabetic neuropathy or structural defects.

Diagnosis of urinary retention following delivery

- Review the case notes for previous and current antenatal history for any risk factors
- Check if labour was prolonged
- Check for epidural use and the last time it was topped up
- Past history of renal or urinary conditions
- Check for a distended bladder, peri-urethral lacerations and vulval haematoma (these can cause severe pain and prevent micturition)

Management of urinary retention

- Foley indwelling catheter for 48 hours if the residual volume is more than 500 ml
- Urine dipstick and MSU if necessary
- Adequate analgesia
- Patient should rarely need self intermittent catheterization
- Urology input in case of any structural defects

Further reading

Collins S, Arulkumaran S, et al. *Oxford Handbook of Obstetrics & Gynaecology*. 3rd ed. Oxford: Oxford University Press; 2013.

20A: False – Most vaginal deliveries are not associated with any problems.
20B: False – Incontinence of flatus or faeces may occur in a minority of women.
20C: True – These factors can also cause anorectal urgency.
20D: False – Pelvic floor denervation may lead to urogenital prolapse. Episiotomy scar or scar from perineal tear both might cause dyspareunia requiring refashioning of the perineum.
20E: True

Preventive measures that may help to avoid pelvic floor damage

- Pelvic floor damage is most likely to occur following a first vaginal delivery.
- Active pushing in the second stage of labour should be limited to around 60 minutes.
- Difficult vaginal and instrumental deliveries should be avoided.
- The damage to the perineum is less with use of vacuum extraction than forceps delivery.
- Pelvic floor exercises are recommended to be started during pregnancy and after delivery.
- An experienced doctor should perform repair of 3rd and 4th degree tears.
- By performing elective caesarean section, the urinary symptoms can be minimized and the coital and anorectal symptoms avoided.

Further reading

Collins S, Arulkumaran S, et al. *Oxford Handbook of Obstetrics & Gynaecology*. 3rd ed. Oxford: Oxford University Press; 2013.

9

POSTPARTUM PROBLEMS (THE PUERPERIUM), INCLUDING NEONATAL PROBLEMS – QUESTIONS

SBAs

Question 1

With respect to postpartum haemorrhage (PPH), which one of the following is the correct statement?

A. The most common cause is retained placenta.
B. Primary PPH is when ≥500 ml of blood loss from the genital tract occurs >48 hours after delivery.
C. Endometritis is a common cause of primary PPH.
D. Routine use of oxytocin in the second stage reduces the risk of postpartum haemorrhage.
E. Prophylactic oxytocics should be offered routinely to all women in the third stage of labour to reduce the risk of postpartum haemorrhage.

Question 2

Neonatal complications of insulin-dependent diabetic mothers include the following except which one?

A. Hypothermia
B. Hyperglycaemia
C. Hypocalcaemia
D. Hypomagnesaemia
E. Respiratory distress syndrome

Question 3

With respect to the fetal circulation, which one of the following is true?

A. Umbilical cord contains two veins and one artery.
B. Umbilical vein carries oxygenated blood from the fetus.
C. Umbilical artery carries deoxygenated blood from the fetus.
D. Umbilical vein carries deoxygenated blood to the fetus.
E. Umbilical artery carries oxygenated blood to the fetus.

Question 4

Which one of the following is incorrect with respect to puerperal pyrexia?

A. Endometritis is a common cause.
B. Puerperal pyrexia refers to a temperature of ≥38°C within the first 6 weeks after delivery.
C. Prolonged rupture of membranes is associated with puerperal pyrexia.
D. Anaemia is a predisposing factor.
E. Mastitis can cause puerperal pyrexia.

Question 5

With respect to puerperal psychosis, which one of the following is true?

A. Unlikely to recur in subsequent pregnancies
B. Characteristically present with manic disorder
C. Occurs in about 1 in 2000 pregnancies
D. Usually occurs about 4 weeks after delivery
E. Puerperal psychosis in a first-degree relative is a risk factor

Question 6

Which one of the following is true regarding neonatal herpes infection?

A. It is associated with less morbidity and mortality.
B. It can be caused by cytomegalovirus.
C. It can be caused either by HSV type 1 or type 2 virus.
D. Most of these infections are due to asymptomatic recurrent herpes virus infection in the mother.
E. It can be caused by hepatitis B virus.

Question 7

With regard to neonatal HSV infection, which one of the following is false?

A. It is a common condition in the UK.
B. It can present with disseminated herpes in the neonate.
C. Infant mortality is decreased with treatment in localized disease of skin, eyes and mouth infection.
D. Disseminated herpes in the neonate is associated with very high mortality if untreated.
E. If treated, disseminated herpes is associated with 30% neonatal mortality.

Question 8

A 29-year-old Asian Indian woman presents to her GP at 39 weeks' gestation with a chickenpox rash of 2 days' duration. She was prescribed oral acyclovir for 7 days and advised not to come in contact with other pregnant women or children. However, 3 days later she presents with spontaneous onset of labour to NHS hospital. She was isolated and barrier nursed. Ten hours later she has a vaginal delivery. What is the appropriate management of the newborn baby in this case?

A. Oral acyclovir
B. Intravenous acyclovir
C. Intravenous varicella immunoglobulin (IVIG)
D. Oral acyclovir and IVIG
E. Intravenous acyclovir and IVIG

EMQs

OPTIONS FOR QUESTIONS 1–3

A. Mastitis
B. Puerperal psychosis
C. Endometritis
D. Retained products of conception
E. Postnatal depression
F. Postpartum blues
G. Breast engorgement
H. Puerperal pyrexia
I. Urinary tract infection
J. Breast abscess

Instructions

For each of the scenarios below, choose the single most appropriate diagnosis from the above list of options. Each option may be used once, more than once or not at all.

1. A 25-year-old parous woman had a spontaneous vaginal delivery followed by retained placenta and manual removal. She attends the emergency department on day 5 postpartum complaining of feeling unwell, heavy bleeding and lower abdominal pains. On examination her pulse is 110, BP 100/70 mm Hg, temperature is 38°C and the uterus is tender with heavy offensive lochia.

2. A 30-year-old para 1 woman was brought in to the hospital 3 weeks after a difficult instrumental delivery as she has been tearful, irritable with lack of interest in herself and her baby. She has been unable to sleep and cope with the demands of the newborn despite family support over the last week.

3. A 34-year-old parous woman with pre-eclampsia at 27 weeks' gestation reported reduced fetal movements and on examination there was no fetal heart. Ultrasound confirmed intrauterine fetal death and a day after the induction of labour she delivered a macerated fetus. On review by the community midwife 3 days later, she was pyrexial with a temperature 37.6°C and both breasts are tender and hard with dilated veins. The abdomen is soft with a non-tender palpable uterus and lochia is normal.

OPTIONS FOR QUESTIONS 4–6

A. Radial nerve palsy
B. Caput succedaneum
C. Erb's palsy
D. Intraventricular haemorrhage
E. Cephalhaematoma
F. Subgaleal haemorrhage
G. Hypoxic ischemic encephalopathy (HIE)
H. Chignon
 I. Subconjunctival haemorrhage
J. Fracture humerus

Instructions

For each of the scenarios below, choose the single most appropriate diagnosis from the above list of options. Each option may be used once, more than once or not at all.

4. A 28-year-old nulliparous woman with a booking BMI of 38 and gestational diabetes on insulin and metformin was induced at 37 weeks' gestation for poor glycaemic control and a big baby. Labour was augmented with syntocinon and she had a forceps delivery for a prolonged second stage, followed by shoulder dystocia. The baby was admitted to the neonatal unit after initial resuscitation and being ventilated. The baby's right arm was noted to be limp with limited movements, but no swelling.

5. A 30-year-old para 1 woman was admitted in spontaneous labour at term and had an emergency caesarean section for failed instrumental delivery. The baby was born in poor condition with low APGARs and was admitted to the neonatal unit after initial resuscitation, where the baby had seizures and was sent for therapeutic cooling.

6. A 30-year-old para 1 woman with previous normal delivery went into spontaneous labour at term and was fully dilated for 3 hours. After pushing for 90 minutes, ventouse delivery was performed for maternal exhaustion and the baby was born in good condition. The parents were extremely anxious after looking at the large soft tissue swelling of the fetal scalp at the ventouse cup application area.

OPTIONS FOR QUESTIONS 7–9

A. Immediate cord clamping
B. Open airway and give 5 inflation breaths
C. Delay cord clamping for at least one minute
D. Chest compressions: 3 inflation breaths to each compression
E. Continue with ventilation breaths
F. Dry the baby
G. Open airway and give 5 ventilation breaths
H. Place in a food-grade plastic bag
I. Chest compressions: 3 compressions to 1 inflation breath
J. Open airway and give 3 inflation breaths

Instructions

For each of the scenarios below, choose the single most immediate plan of action from the above list of options. Each option may be used once, more than once or not at all.

7. A 30-year-old nulliparous woman with no known medical problems had an uncomplicated low-risk pregnancy and went in to spontaneous labour at 39 weeks' gestation. She had good progress in labour and has just delivered a male neonate, who cried at birth, pink, breathing and has good tone.
8. A 33-year-old para 2 woman just delivered a male infant who is blue, floppy at birth with poor respiratory effort and a slow heart rate. The umbilical cord is clamped and cut immediately and placed on the warm resuscitaire after drying and wrapping with warm towels. Baby is gasping and the heart rate is very slow. You call for help and continue with neonatal resuscitation.
9. A 33-year-old para 2 woman just delivered a male infant who is blue, floppy at birth with poor respiratory effort and a slow heart rate. The umbilical cord is clamped and cut immediately and placed on the warm resuscitaire after drying and wrapping with warm towels. You call for help and give two sets of inflation breaths with chin lift. The chest is moving but the heart rate is still <60 beats per minute.

OPTIONS FOR QUESTIONS 10–12

A. Anti-retroviral therapy (ART) should be discontinued
B. ART can be continued
C. Offer 3-yearly cervical cytology
D. Offer hepatitis B and *Varicella zoster* vaccination
E. Offer annual cervical cytology
F. Offer hepatitis B, pneumococcal and influenza vaccination
G. Should be referred for colposcopy
H. No treatment at present
I. Oral acyclovir
J. Offer hepatitis B, mumps and pneumococcal vaccination
K. Commence co-trimoxazole
L. Commence highly active anti-retroviral therapy (HAART)

Instructions

Each clinical scenario described below tests knowledge about the management of women with HIV and their babies. For each one select the single most appropriate management plan. Each option may be used once, more than once or not at all.

10. A 29-year-old woman with a positive HIV test, who was commenced on HAART for prevention of mother to child transmission (PMTCT), has come to see her GP at 28 weeks' gestation to discuss vaccination.
11. A 29-year-old woman taking ART with a plasma viral load greater than 10,000 copies/mL and CD4 lymphocyte counts $500 \times 10^6/l$ has come to the community gynaecology clinic to enquire about cervical screening.
12. A 27-year-old woman had a viral load >1000 HIV RNA copies/mL despite HAART, and the baby was delivered by elective caesarean section at 38 weeks. Which one of the above treatments should the baby receive?

OPTIONS FOR QUESTIONS 13–15

A. Universal antenatal screening for GBS (group B streptococcus)
B. Antenatal oral antibiotics
C. Intrapartum IV benzyl penicillin
D. Intrapartum oral erythromycin
E. No intrapartum antibiotic prophylaxis required
F. Supportive care
G. Repeat testing
H. Treat infection
I. Treat infection as well as intrapartum antibiotics
J. Antibiotics to the newborn

Instructions

Each clinical scenario described below tests knowledge about management of a woman in labour and/or postnatally. For each case, choose the single most appropriate course of action from the above list. Each option may be used once, more than once, or not at all.

13. A 36-year-old woman in her second pregnancy is admitted in early labour with ruptured membranes. She was known to have tested GBS positive in her first pregnancy, but the baby was not affected. She is negative for GBS in this pregnancy.
14. A 34-year-old woman is seen in the antenatal clinic with a history of lower abdominal pain for the past 4 days. She is currently 28 weeks' pregnant and examination reveals closed cervix. Examination of urine confirms colonization with GBS bacteria (greater than 10^5 cfu/ml).
15. A 38-year-old woman attends the antenatal clinic in her second pregnancy. She is currently 16 weeks pregnant. She is very worried about GBS infection and is requesting screening. Her first baby was in a special care baby unit for a prolonged period and treated for neonatal GBS infection.

OPTIONS FOR QUESTIONS 16–18

A. Group B streptococcus (GBS)
B. Group A streptococcus (GAS)
C. Staphylococcal toxic shock syndrome
D. *Clostridium difficile*
E. *Escherichia coli*
F. *Streptococcus pneumoniae*
G. Methicillin-resistant *Staphylococcus aureus* (MRSA)
H. Salmonella
I. Necrotizing fasciitis
J. Gram-negative bacteria

Instructions

Each clinical scenario described below tests knowledge about the most probable cause of sepsis in a woman postnatally. For each case, choose the single most appropriate organism from the above list. Each option may be used once, more than once, or not at all.

16. A 36-year-old woman who had an emergency caesarean section 5 days ago has presented feeling unwell with lower abdominal pain. Examination reveals widespread macular rash and conjunctival hyperaemia. Temperature records 40°C and BP is 90/40 mmHg.
17. A 34-year-old woman had a vaginal delivery 2 days ago. She is seen by the community midwife, who notices that she looks unwell and checks her temperature, which records 39.5°C. The woman is suffering from abdominal pain and loin pain, and was treated for urinary tract infection while pregnant.
18. A 38-year-old woman is brought by ambulance in a state of shock, with sudden-onset lower abdominal pain. She had a baby a week ago and suffered from a recent sore throat, for which she has been taking paracetamol.

MCQs

1. The following are causes of postpartum haemorrhage (PPH):
   A. Vasa praevia
   B. Placenta praevia
   C. Abruption placenta
   D. Atonic uterus
   E. Use of syntocinon after delivery

2. With regard to breastfeeding:
   A. Breastfeeding is contraindicated if the woman has mastitis during the puerperium.
   B. Breastfeeding is contraindicated if the woman has inverted nipples during the puerperium.
   C. Breast milk jaundice usually appears after 7 days of birth.
   D. Breastfeeding is contraindicated if the woman has a breast abscess.
   E. Severe pain is common after regular breastfeeding.

3. The following are causes of puerperal pyrexia:
   A. Breastfeeding
   B. Urinary tract infection
   C. Mastitis
   D. Septic pelvic thromboplebitis
   E. Having episiotomy for assisted delivery

4. Anal incontinence:
   A. Occurs following caesarean section for placenta pravia
   B. Can be caused by perineal trauma during spontaneous vaginal delivery
   C. Can be caused by perineal trauma following forceps delivery
   D. Can be caused by perineal trauma following ventouse delivery
   E. In women does not have an effect on quality of life

5. Newborns with vitamin K deficiency present as follows:
   A. Within first week after birth with umbilical bleeding
   B. Four weeks after birth with rectal bleeding
   C. With circumcision bleeding within first week after birth
   D. With hyperkalaemia
   E. Late onset after one week with signs of bleeding from unusual sites, possibly due to organic pathology

6. Obstetric haemorrhage:
   A. Remains the major cause of maternal death in the UK.
   B. Antepartum haemorrhage is the most common cause of major obstetric haemorrhage in the UK.
   C. In the 2006–08 report of the UK Confidential Enquiries into Maternal Deaths, haemorrhage was the sixth most common cause of maternal death.
   D. The death rate has increased from 3.9 deaths/million maternities in 2003–2005 to 6.6 deaths/million in 2006–2008.
   E. Most deaths due to obstetric haemorrhage in the report were due to substandard care.

7. With regard to chlamydia infection during pregnancy:
   A. It is caused by *Chlamydia trachomatis*.
   B. The reported prevalence in pregnant women is around 7%.
   C. Tetracycline is the drug of choice for treatment of chlamydia during pregnancy.
   D. More than 90% of the neonates born vaginally are colonized with chlamydia in the presence of maternal infection.
   E. Only half of the exposed neonates will develop conjunctivitis in the first 1–2 weeks after birth, in the presence of maternal infection.

8. Regarding anti-D dose and administration following delivery or miscarriage:
   A. It should be administered within 6 hours after vaginal delivery at term.
   B. It should be administered within 72 hours following caesarean section.
   C. If the delivery is at term, the dose of anti-D is 500 IU.
   D. If the delivery is premature, the dose of anti-D is 250 IU.
   E. Anti-D administration is not necessary following a miscarriage after 20 weeks' gestation.

9. Peripartum cardiomyopathy:
   A. Is a common condition
   B. Is associated with increased morbidity and mortality
   C. Is associated with a small heart
   D. Usually occurs in the last month of pregnancy
   E. Is associated with thromboembolism

10. Postpartum psychosis:
    A. Occurs in 2 per 1000 deliveries
    B. Usually presents immediately following delivery
    C. Is usually associated with depression in the postpartum period
    D. Is associated with delusions and hallucinations
    E. Recurs in subsequent pregnancy

11. With regard to the benefits of breastfeeding:
    A. It decreases neonatal immunity.
    B. It increases the incidence of breast cancer.
    C. It promotes uterine contraction and involution of the uterus after delivery.
    D. Partial breast and bottle feeding can be used as lactation amenorrhoea method of contraception
    E. It increases the risk of HIV transmission from mother to baby.

12. With regard to PPH:
    A. The incidence of life threatening PPH occurs in 1 in 10,000 women.
    B. 80–90% of PPH cases are due to uterine atony.
    C. Uterine inversion is the most common cause of PPH.
    D. Uterine rupture is a less common cause of PPH.
    E. Precipitous labour is a risk factor for PPH.

13. The following are true with regard to PPH:
    A. The use of 15-methyl-prostaglandin F2 (haemabate) is contraindicated for use of PPH.
    B. 15-methyl-prostaglandin F2 can be administered intramuscularly in the thigh or buttock.
    C. Ergometrine can be given intramuscularly for quicker action within 1 minute.
    D. Ergometrine should be avoided if possible in women with pre-eclampsia as it can cause sudden increase in blood pressure
    E. If PPH is unresponsive to oxytocin and ergometrine, rectal misoprotol can be used to control PPH.

14. With regard to PPH and signs of hypovolaemia:
    A. Tachycardia occurs when 5% of blood volume is lost.
    B. About 30% of the blood loss causes mild shock with vasoconstriction in the skin and muscles.
    C. Blood loss of 40% or more of blood volume is associated with severe shock affecting heart and brain.
    D. Oliguria is generally seen when blood loss is around 30% of the blood volume.
    E. Paradoxical bradycadia is not a sign of severe hypovolaemia due to haemorrhage.

15. With regard to third-degree perineal tear:
    A. In the UK, clinicians allow 80% of the women to have vaginal delivery after previous tear.
    B. The use of postoperative laxatives is recommended to reduce the incidence of postoperative wound dehiscence.
    C. The ideal suture material for repair of third-degree repair is catgut.
    D. Anal sphincter repair can be performed with vicryl.
    E. Rectovaginal and anovaginal fistulas are common complications of third- and fourth-degree perineal tears.

10

POSTPARTUM PROBLEMS (THE PUERPERIUM), INCLUDING NEONATAL PROBLEMS – ANSWERS

SBAs

Answer 1: E

Primary PPH is defined as the loss of 500 ml or more of blood from the genital tract within 24 hours of birth. The causes of PPH include: tone (uterine atony), trauma (genital tract trauma), tissue (retained placenta) and thrombin (coagulopathy/DIC). Uterine atony is the most common cause, accounting for 70% of cases. Endometritis is the most common cause of secondary PPH. Active management of the third stage of labour lowers maternal blood loss and reduces the risk of PPH. Hence prophylactic oxytocics should be offered to all women routinely in the third stage of labour.

Further reading

RCOG Green-top guideline No. 52. *Prevention and management of postpartum haemorrhage.* 2009. Available at: www.rcog.org.uk /womens-health/clinical-guidance/prevention-and-management -postpartum-haemorrhage-green-top-52

Collins S, Arulkumaran S, et al. *Oxford Handbook of Obstetrics & Gynaecology.* 3rd ed. Oxford: Oxford University Press; 2013.

Answer 2: B

Neonatal complications of diabetic pregnancy include hypoglycaemia, hypocalcaemia, hypomagnesaemia, hypothermia, respiratory distress syndrome, jaundice, polycythaemia, cardiomegaly and birth trauma including shoulder dystocia leading to Erb's palsy, fractures and birth asphyxia.

Further reading

Collins S, Arulkumaran S, et al. *Oxford Handbook of Obstetrics & Gynaecology.* 3rd ed. Oxford: Oxford University Press; 2013.

Answer 3: C

The umbilical cord contains two umbilical arteries and one umbilical vein embedded into the Wharton's jelly. The arteries carry deoxygenated blood from the fetus to the placenta and the umbilical vein carries oxygenated blood to the fetus from the placenta.

Further reading

Collins S, Arulkumaran S, et al. *Oxford Handbook of Obstetrics & Gynaecology.* 3rd ed. Oxford: Oxford University Press; 2013.

Answer 4: B

Puerperal pyrexia is defined as a maternal temperature of ≥38°C maintained over 24 hours or recurring in the first 10 days after childbirth or abortion. Prolonged labour, prolonged rupture of membranes, intrapartum pyrexia, operative delivery, multiple pelvic examinations, episiotomy, vaginal tears, vulvovaginal hematomas and anaemia are predisposing factors.

Further reading

Collins S, Arulkumaran S, et al. *Oxford Handbook of Obstetrics & Gynaecology.* 3rd ed. Oxford: Oxford University Press; 2013.

Maharaj D. Puerperal pyrexia: a review. Part 1. *Obstet Gynecol Surv* 2007; 62:393-399.

RCOG green top guideline no 64B. *Bacterial sepsis following pregnancy.* RCOG; 2012.

Answer 5: E

Puerperal psychosis is a psychiatric emergency, occurring in about 1 in 500 pregnancies and associated with a suicide rate of 5% and an infanticide rate of up to 4%. It usually presents within 2 weeks of delivery and symptoms include delusions, hallucinations, irritable behaviour and suicidal thoughts or thoughts of harming the baby. Most cases are episodes of bipolar affective disorder. The 10-year recurrence rate is up to 80%.

Further reading

Collins S, Arulkumaran S, et al. *Oxford Handbook of Obstetrics & Gynaecology.* 3rd ed. Oxford: Oxford University Press; 2013.

Answer 6: C

Neonatal herpes is rare but associated with a high morbidity and mortality rate. It can be caused by either type 1 or type 2 HSV. Most of the cases are due to HSV type 2 and almost all cases of neonatal herpes occur as a result of direct contact with infected secretions, although cases of postnatal transmissions have been described.

Further reading

Collins S, Arulkumaran S, et al. *Oxford Handbook of Obstetrics & Gynaecology*. 3rd ed. Oxford: Oxford University Press; 2013.

Answer 7: A

Neonatal herpes is rare in the UK. Active surveillance by the British Paediatric Surveillance Unit reported an incidence of 1:60,000 live births annually.

The risks to the fetus can be divided into three types:

1. Infection localized to skin, eyes and mouth
2. Local CNS disease (encephalitis)
3. Disseminated infection with multiple organ involvement

Infant mortality is <2% with treatment in localized skin, eye and mouth infection. In disseminated herpes in the newborn mortality is around 30% if treated with antiviral treatment. Long-term neurological sequel is seen in 17% of cases.

Further reading

RCOG Green-top guideline No. 30. *Genital herpes in pregnancy, management.* 2007. Available at: www.rcog.org.uk/womens-health/clinical-guidance /management-genital-herpes-pregnancy-green-top-30

British Paediatric Surveillance Unit. Available at: www.rcpch.ac.uk/bpsu

Collins S, Arulkumaran S, et al. *Oxford Handbook of Obstetrics & Gynaecology*. 3rd ed. Oxford: Oxford University Press; 2013.

Answer 8: C

If maternal infection occurs at term, there is a significant risk of varicella of the newborn. Ideally elective delivery should normally be avoided until 5–7 days after the onset of maternal rash to allow for the passive transfer of antibodies from the mother to the fetus.

In this case, this woman presents with spontaneous onset of labour and has delivered within 7 days of onset of chickenpox rash. If the onset of the maternal rash is within 7 days of delivery, then the neonate should be given VZIG due to increased risk of neonatal varicella. The newborn baby should be monitored for signs of infection until 28 days after the onset of maternal infection. If the newborn baby develops neonatal varicella, the treatment would involve intravenous acyclovir following discussion with a neonatologist and virologist.

Postnatally, if there is contact with chickenpox in the first 7 days of life, no intervention is required if the mother is immune (the baby would have received passive immunity from the mother). However, the neonate should be given VZIG if the mother is not immune to varicella or if the neonate delivered prematurely.

Neonatal ophthalmic examination should be organized after birth. Neonatal blood should be sent for VZV IgM antibody and later a follow-up sample should be tested for VZV IgG antibody (after 7 months).

Further reading

RCOG Green-top guideline No. 13. *Chickenpox in pregnancy*. 2007. Available at: www.rcog.org.uk/files/rcog-corp/uploaded-files /GT13ChickenpoxinPregnancy2007.pdf

Collins S, Arulkumaran S, et al. *Oxford Handbook of Obstetrics & Gynaecology*. 3rd ed. Oxford: Oxford University Press; 2013.

EMQs

Answers 1–3

1. C

The most likely diagnosis is endometritis in view of the history, symptoms and signs of high temperature, lower abdominal pains, and uterine tenderness with a heavy offensive lochia.

2. E

Postnatal depression usually occurs within the first 4 to 6 weeks and the symptoms include one or more of the following: tearfulness, irritability, low mood for long durations, lack of interest in herself or her baby, unable to cope and sleep, feeling guilty, thoughts of harming herself or baby. History of delusions or hallucinations will indicate psychosis. Postpartum blues occur between days 3 to 10 after delivery and the symptoms spontaneously resolve within a few days without any treatment. Symptoms can include brief episodes of mood lability, tearfulness, poor sleep and irritability; reassurance and support are the mainstay of management.

3. G

If suppression of lactation is not done with bromocriptine-related preparations in women with intrauterine fetal death or stillbirths, breast engorgement occurs during the first day or two. The breasts become tender, firm and distended with dilated veins. Fever can occur in about 15% of women. Supportive measures and expression of breast milk are the mainstays of treatment while lactation suppression becomes effective.

Further reading

Collins S, Arulkumaran S, et al. *Oxford Handbook of Obstetrics & Gynaecology.* 3rd ed. Oxford: Oxford University Press; 2013.

Answers 4–6

4. C

Brachial plexus injury is one of the most important complications of shoulder dystocia though its overall incidence is low. Other fetal complications associated with shoulder dystocia include fractures of the humerus and clavicle, pneumothoraces and hypoxic brain damage.

Further reading

RCOG Green-top guideline No. 42. *Shoulder dystocia.* 2012. Available at: www.rcog .org.uk/files/rcog-corp/GTG42_25112013.pdf

5. G

Asphyxia is a state where placental or pulmonary gas exchange is compromised resulting in cardiorespiratory depression. HIE is a neonatal condition when brain injury occurs as a result of perinatal asphyxia. Therapeutic neonatal hypothermia, where the body temperature is lowered to 33–34°C for 72 hours, is beneficial in reducing the rate of neurodevelopmental disability in survivors.

Further reading

Azzopardi DV, Strohm B, et al. TOBY Study Group. Moderate hypothermia to treat perinatal asphyxial encephalopathy. *N Engl J Med.* 2009; 361:1349–58.

6. H

Chignon is the well-recognized mound of scalp tissue and oedema formed at ventouse delivery as the fetal scalp is drawn into the ventouse cup during the creation of vacuum.

Further reading

Collins S, Arulkumaran S, et al. *Oxford Handbook of Obstetrics & Gynaecology.* 3rd ed. Oxford: Oxford University Press; 2013.

Answers 7–9

7. C

For uncompromised babies, a delay in cord clamping of at least one minute from the complete delivery of the infant is recommended by the neonatal resuscitation council.

8. B

9. I

Further reading

Resuscitation Council (UK). *Neonatal resuscitation guidelines.* 2010. Available at: www.resus.org.uk/pages/nls.pdf

Answers 10–12

10. F

Hepatitis B and pneumococcal vaccination is recommended for all individuals who are HIV positive, and it can be safely administered in pregnancy. Influenza vaccination can also be safely administered in pregnancy and the decision to immunize depends on the time of year. *Varicella zoster* and measles, mumps and rubella vaccines are contraindicated in pregnancy.

11. E

All women who are HIV positive are recommended to have annual cervical cytology; ideally outside pregnancy.

12. K

Pneumocystis pneumonia (PCP) prophylaxis, with co-trimoxazole, should be initiated from age 4 weeks in:

- HIV-positive infants;
- infants with an initial positive HIV DNA/RNA test result (and continued until HIV infection has been excluded); and
- infants whose mother's VL at 36 weeks' gestational age or at delivery is >1000 HIV RNA copies/mL despite HAART or unknown (and continued until HIV infection has been excluded).

Further reading

RCOG Green-top guideline No. 39. *Management of HIV in pregnancy*. 2010. Available at: www.rcog.org.uk/womens-health/clinical-guidance /management-hiv-pregnancy-green-top-39

British HIV Association guidelines. *Management of HIV infection in pregnant women*. 2012. Available at: www.bhiva.org/PregnantWomen2012.aspx

Answers 13–15

13. E
14. I
15. C

- Group B streptococcus is recognized as the most frequent cause of severe early onset (at less than 7 days of age) infection in newborn infants.
- The incidence of early onset GBS disease in the UK in the absence of systematic screening or widespread intrapartum antibiotic prophylaxis (IAP) is 0.5/1000 births, which is similar to that seen in the USA after universal screening and IAP, despite comparable vaginal carriage rates.
- The UK National Screening Committee for the prevention of early onset GBS disease recommended that routine screening using bacteriological culture should not be introduced into UK practice.
- Current evidence does not support screening for GBS or the administration of IAP to women in whom GBS carriage was detected in a previous pregnancy.
- GBS bacteriuria is associated with a higher risk of chorioamnionitis and neonatal disease.
- Women with GBS urinary tract infection during pregnancy should receive appropriate treatment at the time of diagnosis as well as IAP.
- IAP should be offered to women with a previous baby with neonatal GBS disease. Vaginal or rectal swabs are not helpful, as IAP would be recommended even if these swabs were negative for GBS.

Further reading

RCOG Green-top guideline No. 36. *The prevention of early-onset neonatal group B streptococcal disease.* 2012. Available at: www.rcog.org.uk /womens-health/clinical-guidance/prevention-early-onset-neonatal-group-b-streptococcal-disease-green-top-36

Answers 16–18

16. C
17. J
18. B

- NSAIDs significantly impede the ability of polymorphs to fight infection caused by GAS; they should be avoided for pain relief in cases of sepsis.
- Any widespread rash suggests early toxic shock syndrome, especially if conjunctival hyperaemia or suffusion is present.
- Gram-negative bacterial infections are particularly associated with the urinary tract. Acute pyelonephritis should be treated aggressively.
- A history of recent sore throat or prolonged (household) contact with family members with known streptococcal infections (pharyngitis, impetigo, cellulitis) has been implicated in cases of GAS sepsis. In the CMACE report, five of six women with GAS admitted to hospital with septic shock had a history of recent sore throat or respiratory infection.

Further reading

RCOG Green-top guideline No. 64b. *Bacterial sepsis following pregnancy.* 2012. Available at: www.rcog.org.uk/womens-health/clinical-guidance /sepsis-following-pregnancy-bacterial-green-top-64b

MCQs

1A: False – This is bleeding from the fetal vessels.
1B: True
1C: True
1D: True
1E: False

PHH can be either primary or secondary. Primary PPH is defined as blood loss more than 500 ml or more within 24 hours following delivery. Secondary PPH is defined as any excessive bleeding after the first 24 hours following delivery.

Primary PPH

Primary PPH has been one of the major causes of maternal mortality reported during 2000–2002 Confidential Enquiries into Maternal and Child Health (CEMACH) report.
The risk factors for primary PPH include:

- increased maternal age
- increased maternal parity
- twin pregnancy
- obesity
- macrosomic fetus
- antepartum haemorrhage
- previous postpartum haemorrhage
- prolonged labour
- operative vaginal or abdominal delivery

The main causes of primary PPH are:

- uterine atony (90% of cases)
- retained placenta
- retained bits of placenta or membranes
- placenta accrete and praevia
- genital tract trauma during delivery
- coagulopathy

The aide memoire to remember is 4Ts:

- Tone: atony
- Tissue: retained tissue
- Trauma: genital trauma
- Thrombin: coagulation disorder

Secondary PPH

The most common cause of secondary PPH is retained products. The other causes include:

- bleeding from caesarean section incision
- bleeding from placental bed
- hydatidiform mole
- choriocarcinoma
- uterine artery malformations

If the bleeding is related to molar pregnancy, advice from a regional trophoblastic centre should be sought (Charing Cross, Sheffield and Dundee in the UK).

Further reading

Harper A. Massive obstetric haemorrhage. Harper A (ed). *Haemorrhage and Thrombosis for the MRCOG and Beyond*. London: RCOG Press; 2005.

Confidential Enquiries into Maternal and Child Health (CEMACH). *Why Mothers Die 2000–2002. The Sixth Report on the Confidential Enquiries into Maternal Deaths in the United Kingdom*. London: RCOG Press; 2004.

2A: False – Mastitis is not a contraindication for breastfeeding. Regular emptying by breastfeeding on the affected side will improve mastitis sooner.
2B: False – Inverted nipple is not a contraindication for breastfeeding.
2C: False – One should differentiate between breastfeeding jaundice and breast milk jaundice. Breastfeeding jaundice is more of a mechanical problem and is due to insufficient intake of breast milk leading to accumulation of bilirubin in the body due to inadequate bowel movements in the newborn. This can be treated by regular, frequent breastfeeding. On the other hand, breast milk jaundice is a biochemical problem and tends to run in families. It occurs equally in both male and female babies. It may be caused by factors in the breast milk that can block certain proteins in the liver that metabolize bilirubin. These babies may need phototherapy and formula feeds to get their bilirubin levels to normal range
2D: True – Breast abscess should be drained and treated first. However, the woman can breastfeed from the opposite breast.
2E: False – One should check for mastitis if the woman has severe pain in the breast. If this condition persists, lactiferous ducts can become infected and may lead to an abscess formation and sepsis. Therefore, one should not delay giving antibiotics in the presence of symptoms of pain, raised temperature or signs of mastitis (red, tender and swollen breasts).

Further reading

A.D.A.M. Medical Encyclopedia. *Breast milk jaundice*. 2011. Available at: www.ncbi. nm.nih.gov/pubmedhealth/PMH0001990

3A: False
3B: True
3C: True
3D: True

3E: False

The development of fever during the puerperium is a relatively common complication. Although the primary source of this fever usually stems from the genital tract, a thorough evaluation of the febrile puerperal patient for other sites of infection is necessary before initiating antibiotic therapy. Puerperal pyrexia is commonly defined as a temperature elevation of 38°C on two occasions after the first 24 hours following delivery.

Causes of puerperal pyrexia

- Uterine infection
- Infection of abdominal wounds (LSCS)
- Infection of vulval wounds (episotomy or perineal tears)
- Urinary tract infection
- Chest infection
- Mastitis
- Breast abscess
- Septic pelvic vein thromboplebitits
- Ovarian vein thrombosis
- Any abscesses
- Pelvic and vulvovaginal haematoma

Uterine infection

Endometritis is the most common serious complication of the puerperium. Major risk factors for developing postpartum uterine infection include chorioamniotis and abdominal delivery. Other risk factors include prolonged rupture of membranes and multiple cervical examinations. It is commonly caused by *Escherichia coli*, streptococcus A, B or D.

Diagnosis and treatment

Uterine tenderness, offensive vaginal discharge and raised temperature (38°C or more) may all suggest a uterine infection. It is usually a polymicrobiol infection and responds well to antibiotic therapy. Early involvement of microbiologists is invaluable in severely ill patients and those who fail to respond to initial treatment. Metritis in the presence of retained products of conception warrants prompt evacuation. Intravenous antibiotics are continued until the patient has been apyrexial for at least 24 hours.

Endometritis is higher among women who have had caesarean section compared to those who had a vaginal delivery. It is an important cause of maternal morbidity after caesarean section. Prophylactic antibiotic therapy reduces the risk by approximately 60%. The benefit of antibiotic therapy for labouring women has been established. For non-labouring patients, there is still some uncertainty.

Perineal or episiotomy wound infection

Women with this condition can present with fever, discharge from the perineal wound and perineal pain, an inability to pass urine due to severe pain. One should examine the perineum and take swabs for culture and sensitivity prior to treating with antibiotics.

Infection of abdominal wounds (LSCS)

Inspection of the abdominal wounds for any swelling, cellulitis and discharge from the wound is important in the postpartum period. In the presence of a wound discharge, swabs for bacterial culture should be undertaken and antibiotics started. A microbiologist should be involved at the earliest opportunity.

Urinary tract infection

Urinary tract infections (UTIs) are the most frequent nosocomial infections in women during puerperium. Contamination by catheterization, urinary retention and symptomatic bacteriuria all contribute to cystitis. An uncontaminated, catheterized specimen that shows pyuria and bacteriuria will help to make a diagnosis. Treatment with antibiotics should result in prompt resolution of the infection in most cases.

Breast disorders

Various minor breast conditions are common during the puerperium; these include sore nipples, milk stasis and mastitis. More serious examples include abscesses and neoplasms. Inflammatory changes are easily treated with frequent breast emptying; infectious conditions require antibiotics. The symptoms of mastitis are fever, malaise, erythema and pain. The patient is usually several weeks postpartum when this condition develops. *Staphylococcus aureus* and *Staphylococcus epidermidis* are the most common causative organisms. Breast abscesses typically develop in lactating women. Breast abscess need to be ruled out in patients who do not respond to antibiotic treatment. The standard treatment is surgical incision, breaking down of loculi and drainage of pus under antibiotic cover.

Ovarian vein thrombosis

Ovarian vein thrombosis is a rare but potentially serious complication following childbirth. It is difficult to diagnosis and therefore a high index of suspicion is important to make a diagnosis. The incidence is about 1/600 deliveries. Most women present during the first week following delivery. They usually present with fever and right lower quadrant abdominal pain and can therefore mimic appendicitis. It is also associated with leucocytosis. Colour Doppler will help to make a diagnosis as will CT scan. The main treatment consists of anticoagulants and antibiotics.

Vulvovaginal and pelvic haematoma

Vulvovaginal hematoma is an uncommon complication following delivery but can be associated with serious morbidity. Good surgical technique and hemostasis are important while repairing perineal tears and episiotomies. One must examine the perineum if there is a significant drop in blood pressure or significant drop in haemoglobin in a puerperal woman. The management includes corrections of hypovolemia, evacuation of the haematoma and secure haemostasis.

Further reading

Hamadeh G, Dedmon C, Mozley, PD. Postpartum fever. *Am Fam Physician*. 1995; 52(2): 531–8.

Olsen CG, Gordon RE Jr. Breast disorders in nursing mothers. *Am Fam Physician*. 1990; 41(5): 1509–16.

4A: False
4B: True
4C: True
4D: True
4E: False

The definition of anal incontinence is any involuntary loss of faeces or flatus, or urge incontinence that adversely affects the woman's quality of life. It is an embarrassing condition and therefore largely under reported. The prevalence of faecal incontinence is between 0.7% and 0.9% in younger age group (<65 years).

The overall risk of obstetric anal sphincter injury is 1% of all vaginal deliveries. Childbirth is the most common cause of anal sphincter injury leading to faecal incontinence. It may occur following a rectal prolapse or in association with a neurological disorder. The prevalence of these symptoms in women who have undergone third- and fourth-degree tear repair ranges between 20–67%. The type of incontinence can be flatus (59%) or leakage of liquid and solid stool (11%) or solid stool (4%) or faecal urgency (26%).

Mechanism of injury

- Direct mechanical injury to anal sphincter (third- and fourth-degree perineal tears)
- Neurological injury (nerve compression from fetal head or neuropathy of pudendal nerve following forceps delivery)
- A combination of the above

Aetiology of anal incontinence

- Spontaneous vaginal delivery
- Forceps delivery
- Ventouse delivery
- Midline episiotomy
- Previous anal sphincter injury
- Mediolateral episiotomy
- Prolonged second stage of labour
- Birth weight of fetus more than 4 kg
- Epidural analgesia
- Malpositions of the fetal head (e.g. occipitoposterior position of the fetus)

Symptoms

Women may present with passage of flatus when socially undesirable, incontinence of liquid stool, incontinence of solid stool, faecal urgency or a need for wearing a pad because of anal symptoms.

Primary measures to prevent anal sphincter injury

- Aim for spontaneous over instrumental delivery
- Use ventouse over forceps delivery (an RCT found clinical third-degree tears in 16% of women with forceps-assisted deliveries, compared with 7% of vacuum-assisted deliveries)
- Use mediolateral episiotomy over midline episiotomy
- Avoid routine use of episiotomy
- Encourage antenatal pelvic floor exercises
- Encourage antenatal perineal massage

Caesarean sections performed after the onset of labour may not protect the pelvic floor. Elective caesarean section is the only true primary prevention strategy for childbirth injuries to the pelvic floor. However, the effect is nullified after a certain number of caesarean sections.

Secondary measures to prevent anal incontinence

RCOG recommends that all women should have a systematic examination of the perineum, vagina and rectum following vaginal delivery to assess the perineum for damage and extent of damage prior to suturing. Once identified, this should be repaired immediately by an appropriately trained person. Subsequently a follow up should be arranged at 6–12 months for women who had repair of third- and fourth-degree tear.

Tertiary measures to improve quality of life

Symptomatic women at postnatal follow up should be offered endoanal ultrasonography and anorectal manometry and also should be referred to a colorectal surgeon for consideration of secondary repair of anal sphincter.

Subsequent delivery can aggravate anal incontinence. Therefore, women should be assessed for symptoms and counselled appropriately regarding mode of delivery if they had a third- and fourth-degree tear following previous delivery.

Further reading

RCOG Green-top guideline No. 29. *Management of third- and fourth-degree perineal tears*. 2001. Available at: www.rcog.org.uk/womens-health/clinical-guidance /management-third-and-fourth-degree-perineal-tears-green-top-29

Power D, Fitzpatrick M, O'Herlihy C. Obstetric anal sphincter injury: how to avoid, how to repair: A literature review. *J Fam Pract*. 2006; 55:193–200.

Nelson R, Norton N, Cautley E, et al. Community-based prevalence of anal incontinence. *JAMA*. 1995; 274:559–561.

5A: True
5B: False
5C: True
5D: False
5E: True

Intramuscular vitamin K administration for the newborn

Newborns are prone to vitamin K deficiency and therefore all parents should be offered intramuscular vitamin K prophylaxis for their babies at birth (available as KONAKION MM paediatric, phytomenadione 2 mg/ml). Vitamin K should be administered as a single dose of 1 mg (0.5 ml) intramuscularly as this is the most clinically and cost-effective method of administration (NICE 2006). It should be administered into the bulkiest part of the thigh (vastus lateralis thigh muscle, which is located in the front upper outer segment of the thigh in infants). Injection into the buttocks is not recommended, so as to avoid nerve damage.

Oral vitamin K administration for the newborn

If there is a contraindication to intramuscular administration or if the parents decline this route, administration by oral route should be offered. Oral vitamin K dose is 2 mg but in multiple doses. The first dose is after delivery or within 24 hours after birth. The second and third dose would be at 1 week and 6 weeks, respectively. The mother can be discharged home with a prescription for the second dose and for the third dose they should see the GP.

Vitamin K deficiency in the newborn and symptoms

Vitamin K deficiency in the newborn can present within 24 hours (early onset) with bleeding typically from different sites, which include umbilical, oral, rectal and recent circumcision (within one week of birth). Sometimes they can present one week after birth. Often these are due to organic pathology such as malabsorption or liver disease.

Women who decline vitamin K for their babies should be informed about the increased risk of severe haemorrhage and mortality for their baby.

Further reading

NICE clinical guideline No. 37. *Routine postnatal care of women and their babies.* 2006. Available at: www.nice.org.uk/nicemedia/pdf/CG37NICEguideline.pdf

6A: True
6B: False
6C: True
6D: False
6E: True

- Obstetric haemorrhage remains a major cause of maternal death.
- The death rate has decreased from 6.6 deaths/million maternities in 2003–2005 to 3.9 deaths/million in 2006–2008.

- 67% of deaths due to haemorrhage were attributed to substandard care.
- Postpartum haemorrhage (PPH) is the most common form of major obstetric haemorrhage.
- The incidence of PPH is 2–6% of all births and most PPH have no identifiable risk factors.
- Team approach and guideline use has been recommended to prevent maternal death or morbidity from haemorrhage.

Further reading

Lewis G (ed). *Saving Mothers' Lives: Reviewing Maternal Deaths to Make Motherhood Safer: 2003–2005. The Seventh Report of the Confidential Enquiries into Maternal Deaths in the United Kingdom.* London: CMACE; 2007.

Lewis G (ed). *Saving Mothers' Lives: Reviewing Maternal Deaths to Make Motherhood Safer: 2006–2008. The Eighth Report of the Confidential Enquiries into Maternal Deaths in the United Kingdom.* London: CMACE; 2011.

RCOG Green-top guideline No. 52. *Postpartum haemorrhage, prevention and management.* 2009 (Minor revisions November 2009 and April 2011). Available at: www.rcog.org.uk/womens-health/clinical-guidance /prevention-and-management-postpartum-haemorrhage-green-top-52

7A: True – Chlamydia is an obligate intracellular organism.

7B: True – The prevalence is 2–7% in pregnant women.

7C: False – The drug of choice for treatment during pregnancy is erythromycin for 14 days (tetracycline group of drugs are contraindicated as they cause permanent discolouration of the teeth in fetus. It can also effect the calcification of the bones and cause reduced growth of the bones while the fetus is being exposed, which can be reversible once the medication is stopped).

7D: False – Only half of the neonates born vaginally are colonized with chlamydia in the presence of maternal infection.

7E: True – Also, 10–20% of exposed neonates develop pneumonia in the first 8 weeks after birth.

Further reading

Magowan, B. *Churchill's Pocketbook of Obstetrics and Gynaecology.* 3rd ed. Edinburgh: Churchill Livingstone; 2005.

8A: False – Anti-D should be administered within 72 hours following any type of delivery (vaginal, operative or instrumental delivery or caesarean section) or sensitizing event for successful immunoprophylaxis. If it is not given before 72 hours, every effort should still be made to administer the anti-D IgG, as a dose given within 10 days may provide some protection.

8B: True

8C: True

8D: False – Any time after 20 weeks' gestation, 500 IU of anti-D intramuscularly should be given. Give more anti-D if indicated by the Kleihauer test. Ideally this should be done for all women routinely following delivery.

8E: False – If <20 weeks' gestation, 250 IU of anti-D should be administered intramuscularly in the deltoid muscle. Anti-D immunoglobulin is given to Rh-negative women following any sensitizing event during pregnancy (miscarriage at >12 weeks, medical or surgical termination, ectopic pregnancy, normal delivery and antepartum haemorrhage) and prophylactically at 28 and 32 weeks' gestation during the antenatal period. If the woman has recurrent vaginal bleeding after 12 and 20 weeks' gestation, anti-D IgG should be given at 6-weekly intervals. Anti-D IgG should be considered in non-sensitized RhD-negative women if there is heavy or repeated bleeding or associated abdominal pain, as gestation approaches 12 weeks.

Rationale behind anti-D administration

In the UK, 15% of women are rhesus (Rh) negative. NICE recommends that all women should be screened for antibodies at booking visit during pregnancy.

In 18–27% of cases, late immunization can occur during the third trimester of a first pregnancy. This risk falls to 1% during first pregnancy and 3–5% during subsequent pregnancies, if anti-D is administered. In 10% of cases there is no recognized cause for sensitization. If the father is homozygous for 'D' there is a 100% chance that the fetus is Rh positive, while if he is heterozygous for 'D' there is 50% chance that the fetus will be Rh-positive. However, if the father is homogygous for 'd' then both father and the fetus will be Rh-negative and therefore rhesus disease is said to be unlikely.

Further reading

RCOG Green-top guideline No. 22. *The use of anti-D immunoglobulin for rhesus D prophylaxis.* 2011. Available at: www.rcog.org.uk/womens-health /clinical-guidance/use-anti-d-immunoglobulin-rh-prophylaxis-green-top-22

Magowan, B. *Churchill's Pocketbook of Obstetrics and Gynaecology.* 3rd ed. Edinburgh: Churchill Livingstone; 2005.

9A: False
9B: True
9C: False
9D: True
9E: True

- Peripartum cardiomyopathy is a rare condition.
- It carries a mortality of 25–50%.
- Common in multiparous and of African descent.
- Usually presents after 30 weeks' gestation.
- Heart failure occurs during the last month of pregnancy or within the first 6 months after delivery.
- The presentation is sudden onset of cardiac failure with echocardiogram showing a large dilated heart.
- The following drugs are used in the management of the condition: frusemide, digoxin, nitrates and angiotensin-converting enzyme inhibitors.

- Thromboprophylaxis with heparin is very important to reduce the risk of venous thromboembolism.
- In women presenting during the antenatal period, delivery is indicated.
- The risk of recurrence of peripartum cardiomyopathy in subsequent pregnancies is as high as 85%.

Further reading

Nelson-Piercy, C. *Handbook of Obstetric Medicine*. 4th ed. London: Informa Healthcare; 2010.

10A: True
10B: False
10C: False – Depression is not seen often.
10D: True
10E: True – The risk of recurrence in subsequent pregnancies is around 21–50%.

Difference between Postpartum Blues, Psychosis and Depression

Postpartum blues	Postpartum psychosis
Seen in 50–70% of women	Is uncommon and seen in 2 per 1000 deliveries
Usually manifests in the first few days after delivery	Usually presents after 2–3 days and before 3 weeks after delivery
Cause is multifactorial and seen in all ethnic and social groups	Women give history of bipolar disease in 40% of cases. One should also rule out other organic conditions such as sepsis, electrolyte imbalance, metabolic disturbance and intoxication
Symptoms include tearfulness, lack of sleep, anxiety, headache, poor concentration, fatigue and depression	Symptoms include mania, delusions and hallucinations (auditory commands to harm the baby)
Treatment is reassurance, education and support	Treatment consists of admission of woman to the mother and baby unit. Antipsychotic medication (chlorpromazine or haloperidol). Antidepressants and benzodiazepines may also be necessary. Electroconvulsive therapy has also been used successfully to treat postpartum depression
Postpartum depression	

Postpartum depression affects around 10–14% of women.

Severe depression lasting more than 2 weeks after delivery is suggestive of postpartum depression.

The diagnosis is made when five of the following symptoms (criteria from *DSM-IV*) are present for at least 2 weeks. These include depressed mood, major changes in weight or appetite, anhedonia (lack of enjoyment of life), fatigue, psychomotor agitation, feelings of worthlessness, decreased or lack of concentration, lack of sleep, excessive sleep and recurrent thoughts of death or suicide.

The treatment consists of admission to the mother and baby unit, psychotherapy and pharmacotherapy (SSRIs, tricyclics and lithium). Electroconvulsive therapy has also been used successfully to treat postpartum depression.

Further reading

American Psychiatric Association. *Diagnostic and Statistical Manual of Mental Health Disorders.* 4th ed. (DSM-IV-TR). Arlington: American Psychiatric Publishing Inc.; 1994.

RCOG Good Practice No. 14. *Management of women with mental health issues during pregnancy and the postnatal period.* 2011. Available at: www.rcog .org.uk/management-women-mental-health-issues-during-pregnancy-and -postnatal-period

Magowan, B. *Churchill's Pocketbook of Obstetrics and Gynaecology.* 3rd ed. Edinburgh: Churchill Livingstone; 2005.

James D, Steer PJ, et al. (eds). *High Risk Pregnancy: Management Options.* 4th ed. St Louis: Saunders; 2011.

11A: False – Breastfeeding increases neonatal immunity due to transfer of IgA antibodies and lactoferrin in breast milk.
11B: False – Breastfeeding decreases the risk of breast cancer and this effect is increased with the increase in duration of breastfeeding
11C: True – Suckling stimulates release of oxytocin from the pituitary gland. This causes uterine contraction and promotes uterine involution.
11D: False – Breastfeeding causes release of prolactin from the pituitary and increases the serum levels of prolactin. This not only promotes milk production but also has a contraceptive effect as it inhibits ovulation (by inhibiting LH and FSH). Exclusive breastfeeding can be used as lactation amenorrhoea method for contraception. If breastfeeding is not the sole method of feeding the baby, alternative contraception should be used.
11E: True – It increases vertical transmission. Women are advised to bottlefeed their babies.

Further reading

Collins S, Arulkumaran S, et al. *Oxford Handbook of Obstetrics & Gynaecology.* 3rd ed. Oxford: Oxford University Press; 2013.

12A: False – Life threatening, occurs in 1 in 1000 women.
12B: True
12C: False – Uterine inversion is a less common cause of PPH.
12D: True
12E: True

Further reading

Collins S, Arulkumaran S, et al. *Oxford Handbook of Obstetrics & Gynaecology.* 3rd ed. Oxford: Oxford University Press; 2013.

13A: False – PPH can be treated with 15-methyl-prostaglandin F2 (haemabate). Haemabate (250 mcg IM) can be repeated at 15-minute intervals for a maximum of 8 doses.

13B: True

13C: False – Ergometrine can be administered by both intramuscular and intravenous route. For quicker action within 1 minute, it should be used intravenously but at the cost of excessive vomiting (side effect of ergometrine).

13D: True

13E: True – Rectal misoprotol (1000 mcg) can be used for this purpose. It mainly causes GI side effects (diarrhoea).

Further reading

Collins S, Arulkumaran S, et al. *Oxford Handbook of Obstetrics & Gynaecology.* 3rd ed. Oxford: Oxford University Press; 2013.

14A: False – Tachycardia occurs when 15–30% blood volume is lost.

14B: True – The woman can feel weak and appear pale at this stage.

14C: True – Symptoms related to the compromise of blood supply to the brain and heart can be evident at this stage.

14D: True – Vasoconstriction to splanchnic and renal vessels occur at this stage and leads to oliguria.

14E: False – Bradycardia should not be ignored as normal as this can be a sign of severe hypovolaemia.

Further reading

Collins S, Arulkumaran S, et al. *Oxford Handbook of Obstetrics & Gynaecology.* 3rd ed. Oxford: Oxford University Press; 2013.

15A: True – There is no evidence that the incidence of third-degree perineal tear is reduced if caesarean section is performed in women with previous third-degree perineal tear.

15B: True – It should be performed by an experienced clinician, under good light, under regional or general anaesthesia to enable adequate retraction of the torn ends of the anal sphincter.

15C: False – Catgut has a short half-life and is absorbed very quickly and therefore not suitable for anal sphincter repair. Catgut is no longer in use in UK after the BSE (bovine spongiform encephalopathy) problem. The ideal suture material is PDS (delayed absorbable suture) but vicryl can also be used.

15D: True

15E: False – Both rectovaginal and anovaginal fistulas are rare complications of these perineal tears and occur in less than 5% of repairs.

Further reading

RCOG Green-top guideline No. 29. *Third- and fourth-degree perineal tears, management.* 2007. Available at: www.rcog.org.uk /womens-health/clinical-guidance/management-third-and -fourth-degree-perineal-tears-green-top-29

Collins S, Arulkumaran S, et al. *Oxford Handbook of Obstetrics & Gynaecology.* 3rd ed. Oxford: Oxford University Press; 2013.

GYNAECOLOGICAL PROBLEMS – QUESTIONS

SBAs

Question 1

Which one of the following statements is false with regard to the human papilloma virus (HPV)?

A. HPV type 6 and type 11 are the commonest cause of anogenital warts.
B. HPV type 16 and type 18 are oncogenic.
C. HPV 16 and 18 are associated with up to 75% of cervical cancers.
D. Gardasil vaccine protects against types 6, 11, 16, and 18.
E. Cervarix vaccine protects against genital warts.

Question 2

Which one of the following is true with regard to the cervical screening programme in the UK?

A. Cervical screening starts at the age of 20 years in England.
B. Cervical screening is a test for cervical cancer.
C. All women between the ages of 20 and 65 years should be screened every 3 years.
D. Liquid-based cytology is more cost effective than the traditional Pap smear test.
E. Cervical screening is not necessary if a woman has never been sexually active.

Question 3

Which one of the following is not a procedure for the surgical treatment of stress continence?

A. Colposuspension
B. Synthetic mid-urethral tapes
C. Botulinum injection to bladder
D. Autologous rectus fascial sling
E. Intramural bulking agent injection

Question 4

With respect to the management of female urinary incontinence, which one of the following statements is incorrect?

A. For women with stress incontinence, supervised pelvic floor muscle training for at least 3 months duration is the recommended first-line treatment.
B. Pelvic floor muscle training should consist of at least 8 contractions performed three times a day.
C. The recommended first-line treatment for women with urge incontinence is bladder training for at least 6 weeks.
D. Pelvic floor muscle training in combination with electrical stimulation is more effective and should be routinely offered to women with overactive bladder.
E. Bladder diaries should be used in the initial assessment of women with urinary incontinence.

Question 5

With regard to Turner syndrome the following statements are true except which one?

A. It may present with menorrhagia.
B. It is associated with gonadal dysgenesis.
C. It has karyotype 45XO.
D. It is associated with coarctation of aorta.
E. It is possible to conceive and have children.

Question 6

With regard to CIN and cervical cancer, which one of the following statements is correct?

A. The incidence of cervical cancer is increasing in the UK.
B. The mortality rate due to cervical cancer is increasing in the UK.
C. The incidence of inadequate smears is around 50%.
D. The sensitivity of cervical cytology is 100%.
E. Despite a good screening programme, a negative smear does not provide 100% protection against cervical cancer.

Question 7

Which one of the following statements with regard to CIN is true?

A. CIN 1 progression to invasive cancer is quicker than CIN 2 and CIN 3.
B. CIN 1 always needs treatment when detected on colposcopy.
C. CIN 1 will need treatment if persistent for long time.
D. CIN 2 and 3 can be left for 2 years before treatment.
E. Almost 90% of low-grade cytological abnormalities that are not treated at a first visit will revert to normal cytology and colposcopy.

Question 8

With regard to cervical glandular intraepithelial neoplasia (CGIN), which one of the following statements is correct?

A. Cervical smear is designed to pick up these abnormalities easily.
B. It is a malignant glandular lesion of the cervix.
C. The incidence of CGIN in cervical cytology is 1%.
D. 80% of CGIN are associated with CIN.
E. CGIN is difficult to treat as it is associated with skip lesions higher up in the canal.

Question 9

Which one of the following statements about vulval intraepithelial neoplasia (VIN) is true?

A. The incidence of VIN is decreasing in younger women.
B. VIN can be associated with uterine cancer.
C. VIN can progress to vulval cancer.
D. VIN is always secondary to HPV infection.
E. VIN is always a multifocal disease.

Question 10

Which one of the following is true regarding tamoxifen?

A. It acts as an oestrogen agonist on breast tissue.
B. It acts as an oestrogen antagonist on endometrium.
C. It can be used for ovulation induction.
D. It is not associated with endometrial hyperplasia.
E. It is not associated with endometrial cancer.

Question 11

The following cancers are correctly matched with their respective tumour marker except which one?

A. Inhibin B – Granulosa cell tumour
B. CA 19.9 – Epithelial ovarian cancer
C. Alphafetoprotein (AFP) – Endodermal sinus tumour of the ovary
D. Oestradiol – Granulosa cell tumour
E. CA 15.3 – Breast cancer

EMQs

OPTIONS FOR QUESTIONS 1–3

A. Diuretic-induced leak
B. Detrusor overactivity
C. Incontinence due to neurological damage
D. Mixed incontinence
E. Overflow incontinence
F. Urge incontinence
G. Stress incontinence
H. Recto-vaginal fistula
I. Urgency
J. Urinary tract infection
K. Uretero-vaginal fistula
L. Vesico-vaginal fistula
M. Vesico-sigmoid fistula

Instructions

For each clinical scenario described below, choose the single most likely diagnosis from the list above. Each answer can be used once, more than once or not at all.

1. A 48-year-old woman presents with incontinence of urine. She is hypertensive and is on bendroflumethiazide. She is reviewed by her GP and is referred for pelvic floor exercises. Three months later she is again reviewed by GP but the symptoms have not improved. She is therefore referred for urodynamic testing, which shows leak on coughing.
2. A 30-year-old woman presents with increased frequency of micturition to the maternity day assessment unit. Her urine dipstick is positive for proteins, ketones and nitrates. She had caesarean section for prolonged second stage of labour 5 days ago, in a different hospital.
3. A 49-year-old woman presents with frequency, urgency and urge incontinence. She gets up in the night at least three times to pass urine and has disturbed sleep. She is referred for urodynamics, which shows detrusor contractions during the filling phase.

OPTIONS FOR QUESTIONS 4–6

A. Total abdominal hysterectomy
B. Endometrial ablation
C. Out-patient hysteroscopy + endometrial biopsy
D. Vaginal hysterectomy
E. No intervention required
F. Hysteroscopy + endometrial biopsy + Mirena IUS
G. Total abdominal hysterectomy + bilateral salpingo-oophorectomy
H. Myomectomy
 I. Transcervical resection of fibroid
J. Uterine artery embolization

Instructions

For each clinical scenario below, choose the single most appropriate surgery from the above list of options. Each option may be used once, more than once or not at all.

4. A 47-year-old multiparous woman with known fibroids attends the gynaecology clinic with a history of heavy periods with flooding and clots. She is symptomatic with anaemia and has pressure symptoms. On examination, the uterus is 28 weeks' size and freely mobile. Multiple large fundal and posterior wall intramural fibroids, but no submucous fibroids, were reported on ultrasound. Endometrial sampling showed secretary endometrium with no evidence of inflammation or hyperplasia. She has completed her family.

5. A 50-year-old para 3 woman attends the gynaecology clinic with a history of fullness and a dragging sensation in the vagina. Her menstrual cycles are irregular with heavy and prolonged bleeding for 6 months, not responding to medical treatment. On examination there is grade two utero-vaginal prolapse with mild cystocele. The uterus is bulky and both ovaries appear normal on ultrasound. Endometrial biopsy shows a normal proliferative endometrium with no evidence of inflammation, hyperplasia or malignancy.

6. A 58-year-old para 2 woman was referred to the gynaecology clinic after one episode of postmenopausal bleeding. There is no history of post-coital bleeding. She is not on hormone replacement therapy and her cervical smear is normal. Pelvic ultrasound shows a normal uterus with an endometrial thickness of 6 mm and normal ovaries.

OPTIONS FOR QUESTIONS 7–9

A. Repeat semen analysis immediately
B. Laparoscopy and dye test
C. Serum progesterone on day 28 and then weekly until next cycle
D. Hysterosalpingography (HSG)
E. Serum follicle-stimulating hormone
F. Serum estradiol
G. Antisperm antibody screening
H. Hysterosalpingo-contrast-ultrasonography
I. Serum progesterone on day 21
J. Repeat semen analysis in 3 months after the initial test

Instructions

For each clinical scenario below, choose the single most appropriate intervention from the above list of options. Each option may be used once, more than once or not at all.

7. A 28-year-old woman with a previous ectopic pregnancy and endometriosis has been trying to conceive for more than 18 months. Her GP has initiated the investigations for the couple and the hormonal profile, pelvic ultrasound and semen analysis were normal. You would like to establish the tubal patency.

8. A 30-year-old nulliparous woman attends with her 40-year-old partner for a follow-up fertility clinic appointment. They were referred with a history of primary subfertility and all the baseline investigations were requested at the initial visit. Semen analysis results are as follows: semen volume, 3 ml; sperm concentration, 12 million/ml; total sperm number, 36 million; normal forms, >30%; normal motility, 60%; progressive motility, 40%.

9. A 28-year-old woman with a BMI of 38 attends the fertility clinic with a history of primary subfertility. Her menstrual cycles were irregular once in every 35 to 60 days but she has had 35-day cycles during the last 3 months. You would like to establish the ovulation status of these cycles and ask her to do one of the above tests.

OPTIONS FOR QUESTIONS 10–12

A. Stress incontinence
B. Urge incontinence
C. Vesico-vaginal fistula
D. Mixed incontinence
E. Interstitial cystitis
F. Detrusor overactivity
G. Overactive bladder syndrome (OAB)
H. Overflow incontinence
 I. Urinary urgency
 J. Urodynamic stress incontinence

Instructions

For each clinical scenario below, choose the single most appropriate diagnosis from the options list. Each option may be used once, more than once or not at all.

10. A 25-year-old para 1 woman reports leakage of urine on the postnatal ward on day 2 post delivery. She had a prolonged labour due to slow progress in the first stage, oxytocin augmentation, epidural analgesia and forceps delivery for prolonged second stage followed by a third-degree tear repair. The catheter was removed >12 hours ago and she passed small amounts of urine on few occasions since then.
11. A 50-year-old woman complains of urinary leakage on coughing, sneezing, laughing and any exertion. She has made lifestyle changes, lost weight and has been doing pelvic floor exercises for the last 9 months with minimal symptomatic improvement. Urodynamic studies confirmed the diagnosis and insertion of a synthetic mid-urethral tape procedure is organized.
12. A 65-year-old woman complains of urinary frequency, urgency, nocturia and urge incontinence. Urodynamic investigations show involuntary detrusor contractions during the filling phase of the micturition cycle. She has made lifestyle changes, bladder training and is happy with the symptomatic improvement with anticholinergic medication.

OPTIONS FOR QUESTIONS 13–15

A. Pelvic floor muscle training of at least 3 months
B. Sacrocolpopexy
C. Bladder training for 6 months
D. Botulinum toxin injection
E. Bladder training for 3 months
F. Pelvic floor muscle training of at least 6 months
G. Transobturator tape insertion
H. Bladder training for 6 weeks
I. Pelvic floor muscle training of at least 6 weeks
J. Cystoscopy

Instructions

For each of the scenarios below, choose the single most appropriate intervention from the above list of options. Each option may be used once, more than once or not at all.

13. A 42-year-old para 1 woman complains of urinary leakage on coughing, sneezing, laughing and any exertion. She has no urinary frequency, urgency or urge leaks. Urodynamic studies confirm stress incontinence with no evidence of detrusor overactivity. As per NICE guidelines, the first-line treatment is a trial of supervised training of one of the above.

14. A 65-year-old para 2 woman complains of urinary frequency, urgency, nocturia and urge leaks with occasional stress leaks on exertion. There is no evidence of urinary tract infection. She has made lifestyle changes and urodynamic studies confirm detrusor overactivity. As per NICE guidelines, the first-line treatment for her is a trial of supervised training of one of the above.

15. A 48-year-old para 2 woman was diagnosed with urodynamic stress incontinence more than a year ago and had minimal symptomatic improvement despite lifestyle changes, weight loss and regular pelvic floor muscle exercises. She is keen to have a surgical procedure and is booked to have one of the above procedures.

OPTIONS FOR QUESTIONS 16–18

A. Appendicitis
B. Ovarian cyst accident
C. Ectopic pregnancy
D. Urinary tract infection
E. Ureteric colic
F. Acute pelvic inflammatory disease
G. Haemorrhagic corpus luteum
H. Mittlesmertz
I. Endometriosis
J. Diverticulitis

Instructions

For each of the clinical scenarios below, choose the single most likely diagnosis from the above list of options. Each option may be used once, more than once or not at all.

16. A 24-year-old woman presents to the emergency department with a 6-hour history of severe right lower abdominal pain and nausea. Her last menstrual period was 5 weeks ago. On examination there is tenderness in the right iliac fossa, but no guarding or rebound tenderness. Her pulse is 92 and BP 120/60 mmHg. Her Hb is 14 gm/dl, WBC 8×10^6, CRP 5. Urine hCG is positive.

17. A 26-year-old woman presents to the emergency department with a 6-hour history of right lower abdominal pain and nausea. Her last menstrual period was 2 weeks ago. On examination there is tenderness in the suprapubic and right and left iliac fossae with guarding and rebound tenderness. On speculum examination, there is minimal discharge. Her Hb is 13.6 gm/dl, WBC 22×106, CRP is 70. Pulse is 96, BP 130/80 mmHg and temperature is 38.6°C. Urine hCG is negative. Pelvic ultrasound shows normal pelvic organs with minimal free fluid in the pouch of Douglas.

18. A 25-year-old woman presents to the emergency department with a 6-hour history of sudden onset of right lower abdominal pain at 14 weeks' gestation. Her pulse is 100, BP is 126/86 mmHg. On examination there is suprapubic and left iliac fossae tenderness with guarding. Her Hb is 13 gm/dl, WBC 13×10^6 and CRP 20. Her dating scan a week ago confirmed normal intrauterine pregnancy and a simple left ovarian cyst measuring 4×5 cm in size.

OPTIONS FOR QUESTIONS 19–21

A. Serum CA-125 testing
B. Serum α-FP and hCG testing in addition to CA-125
C. MRI pelvis
D. Exploratory laparotomy
E. Diagnostic laparoscopy
F. No treatment
G. Combined pill
H. Ovarian cystectomy
I. Oophorectomy
J. Ultrasound surveillance

Instructions

Each clinical scenario described below tests knowledge about management of a woman diagnosed with ovarian cyst. For each case, choose the single most appropriate course of action from the above list. Each option may be used once, more than once or not at all.

19. A 34-year-old woman attends the gynaecology clinic with an ultrasound finding of a 5 cm complex right ovarian mass.
20. A 28-year-old woman, who is referred for irregular periods, has a pelvic ultrasound scan, which reports a 6 cm simple ovarian cyst. There is no evidence of ascites or any suspicious features on the scan and she has no pain.
21. A 35-year-old woman who is investigated for sub-fertility has an ultrasound scan showing a 6 cm ovarian lesion suspicious of endometrioma.

OPTIONS FOR QUESTIONS 22–24

A. Serum CA-125 and pelvic ultrasound
B. Cyst aspiration
C. MRI pelvis
D. Staging laparotomy
E. Diagnostic laparoscopy
F. No treatment
G. Combined pill
H. Ovarian cystectomy
I. Oophorectomy
J. Ultrasound surveillance

Instructions

Each clinical scenario described below tests knowledge about management of a woman diagnosed with an ovarian mass. For each case, choose the single most appropriate course of action from the above list. Each option may be used once, more than once or not at all.

22. A 56-year-old woman has been experiencing intermittent lower abdominal pain and pelvic ultrasound scan reveals a 7 cm simple ovarian cyst on the right. Rest of pelvis is normal and serum CA-125 is low.
23. A 58-year-old woman noticed some postmenopausal bleeding and ultrasound scan and MRI scan revealed a complex left adnexal mass with serum CA-125 100 u/ml.
24. A 52-year-old woman is seen in the community clinic repeatedly with persistent abdominal distension and feeling full. She has been experiencing loss of appetite and mild lower abdominal pain. On enquiry she reports to have noticed increased urinary urgency.

OPTIONS FOR QUESTIONS 25–27

A. Mirena IUS
B. Cyst aspiration
C. Nonsteroidal anti-inflammatory drugs
D. Danazol
E. Diagnostic laparoscopy
F. Supportive care
G. Combined oral contraceptive pill
H. Ovarian cystectomy
I. Oophorectomy
J. GnRH analogue

Instructions

Each clinical scenario described below tests knowledge about management of a woman diagnosed with an ovarian mass. For each case, choose the single most appropriate course of action from the above list. Each option may be used once, more than once or not at all.

25. A 36-year-old woman presents with lower abdominal pain, increasing abdominal distension, shortness of breath and a subjective impression of reduced urine output. She had taken clomiphene citrate for ovulation induction. Pelvic ultrasound scan revealed enlarged ovary with multiple cysts.
26. A 34-year-old woman is seen in the clinic with c/o lower abdominal pain for the past 2 years. The pain is usually noticed at the time of periods and recently she is experiencing some deep dyspareunia. She is not currently contemplating pregnancy and her body mass index (BMI) is 26.
27. A 38-year-old woman is investigated for primary sub-fertility and is awaiting IVF. Her partner's semen analysis was normal. Pelvic ultrasound scan revealed a 5 cm right ovarian cyst suggestive of endometrioma.

MCQs

1. With regard to the management of premenstual syndrome (PMS):
    A. Microgynon (conventional combined oral contraceptive pill) is preferable to a newer COCP (e.g. Yasmin).
    B. Cognitive therapy should not be used for all women with PMS.
    C. Cyclical use of COCP has shown to be more effective than continuous (back-to-back) use.
    D. Selective serotonin-release inhibitors (SSRIs) improve physical but not psychological symptoms.
    E. The evidence for use of complementary therapy is limited.

2. Hormonal replacement therapy (HRT) increases the risk of:
    A. Endometrial cancer
    B. Colon cancer
    C. Lung cancer
    D. Fallopian tube cancer
    E. Bartholin gland cancer

3. Bacterial vaginosis (BV):
    A. Is a sexually transmitted disease
    B. Can be diagnosed by taking a vaginal swab for culture
    C. Is caused by overgrowth of anaerobes in the vagina
    D. Can present with vaginal discharge that typically has a fishy odour
    E. Is caused only by *Gardnerella vaginalis*

4. With regard to human papilloma virus (HPV):
    A. HPV can be sexually transmitted.
    B. HPV infection of the cervix is quite common in women who are less than 25 years of age.
    C. HPV is a single stranded RNA virus.
    D. HPV vaccine can be used to prevent particular HPV infection in women who have been sexually active.
    E. The persistence of HPV infection protects women with developing cervical intraepithelial neoplasia (CIN).

5. Menorrhagia is caused by:
    A. Adenomyosis of the uterus
    B. Subserous fibroids
    C. Endometriosis
    D. Endometrial atrophy
    E. Mirena IUS

6. Secondary amenorrhoea:
    A. Is defined as absence of a menstrual period for 6 months
    B. Is defined as absence of menstrual period equivalent to three previous cycle lengths
    C. Is defined as absence of a menstrual period after the age of 40 years
    D. Is defined as absence of a menstrual period before the age of 40 years
    E. Is defined as absence of a menstrual periods before the age of 8 years

7. Tumour marker CA-125:
   A. Is raised in 80% of stage 1 epithelial ovarian cancer
   B. Is always raised in women with epithelial ovarian cancer
   C. Can be raised in diverticulosis
   D. Can be raised in inflammatory bowel disease
   E. Can be raised in pelvic inflammatory disease

8. Serum testosterone levels:
   A. Can be raised in women with adenomyosis
   B. Can be raised in women with polycystic ovarian syndrome
   C. Can be raised in women with ovarian tumours
   D. Can be raised in women with pelvic endometriosis
   E. Can be raised in women with late-onset congenital adrenal hyperplasia

9. The following tumour markers are raised in dysgerminoma:
   A. CA-125
   B. Carcinoembryonic antigen (CEA)
   C. CA-15.3
   D. CA-19.9
   E. Alpha feto-protein (AFP)

10. The following options can be used in the treatment of hirsutism:
    A. Weight loss
    B. Mechanical epilators
    C. Clomiphene citrate
    D. COCP
    E. Octreotide

11. The following conditions can cause puberty menorrhagia:
    A. Bleeding disorders
    B. Leukemia
    C. Previous splenectomy
    D. Regular monthly ovulation
    E. Thyroid disorders

12. With regard to the treatment of puberty menorrhagia:
    A. First-line treatment is endometrial ablation.
    B. Second-line treatment is hysterectomy.
    C. Third-line treatment is medical.
    D. It can be treated with oral progestogens.
    E. It can be treated with COCP.

13. Dysfunctional uterine bleeding is caused by:
    A. Fibroids
    B. Copper IUD
    C. Endometriosis
    D. Ovarian cyst
    E. Pelvic congestion syndrome

14. The following conditions can cause hirsutism:
    A. Cushing syndrome
    B. Endometrial hyperplasia
    C. Hypothyroidism
    D. Congenital adrenal hyperplasia
    E. Late-onset congenital adrenal hyperplasia

15. A detailed history for hirsutism should include:
    A. Dietary history
    B. Duration of hirsutism
    C. Any associated voice changes
    D. Any history of clitoromegaly
    E. Any changes to menstrual cycle

16. With regard to the investigations and diagnosis of hirsutism:
    A. Testosterone levels are always raised in women with PCOS.
    B. Extremely high levels of 17-OH progesterone are seen in women with PCOS.
    C. Dehydro-epiandrosterone sulphate (DHEAS) is increased in adrenal tumours.
    D. Women with PCOS will have low sex hormone-binding globulin (SHBG) due to increased testosterone levels.
    E. Women with adrenal tumours may have voice changes and clitoromegaly on examination.

17. The drugs used in the treatment of hirsutism include:
    A. Combined oral contraceptive pill (COCP)
    B. Spironolactone
    C. Fluconazole
    D. Finesteride
    E. Haloperidol

18. Pelvic inflammatory disease (PID):
    A. Is ascending infection of the lower genital tract
    B. Is more common after the age of 40 years
    C. Is common in women with previous history of PID
    D. Can be precipitated by uterine instrumentation
    E. Can occur within 3 weeks of insertion of intrauterine (e.g. IUCD) insertion

19. The following are indications for hospitalization in a patient with PID:
    A. Inability to tolerate oral medications
    B. Temperature >38.5°C
    C. Evidence of tubo-ovarian abscess on ultrasound scan
    D. If the woman is taking COCP for contraception
    E. If the woman lives alone at home

20. The long-term sequelae of PID include:
    A. Endometriosis
    B. Vaginal adhesions
    C. Ectopic pregnancy
    D. Psychological trauma
    E. PCOS

21. The following investigations may be required to diagnose a woman with PID:
    A. Serum βhCG
    B. White blood cell count (WBC)
    C. Endocervical swab for Chlamydia
    D. Low vaginal swab (LVS)
    E. Laparoscopy

22. Women with trichomonas infection may present with:
    A. Vulvovaginitis
    B. Dysuria
    C. Thin serous vaginal discharge
    D. Fishy smell of vaginal discharge
    E. Tubo-ovarian abscess

23. The following are true with regard to sexually transmitted infections (STIs):
    A. Chlamydia is really rare in the UK.
    B. Gonorrhoea is the second commonest STI in the UK.
    C. Tricomonas is usually associated with other STIs.
    D. Syphilis is rare in the UK.
    E. *Bacterial vaginosis* is not considered an STI.

24. Syphilis:
    A. Is caused by Haemophylus ducreyi
    B. Has a short incubation period (5–7 days)
    C. Can present with secondary syphilis
    D. Can present with tertiary syphilis
    E. Can present with neurosyphillis

25. With regard to human papilloma virus (HPV) infection:
    A. HPV 18 causes genital warts.
    B. HPV 16 can cause cervical intraepithelial neoplasia.
    C. HPV can cause cervical cancer if the virus persists in cervix.
    D. Women with HPV infection are often symptomatic.
    E. It can resolve by itself in young women.

26. Risk factors for endometrial cancer include:
    A. BRCA1 positive
    B. PCOS
    C. Induction of ovulation with clomiphene citrate
    D. Induction of ovulation with tamoxifen
    E. Hereditary non-polyposis colon cancer (HNPCC)

27. Women going through the menopause experience:
    A. Hot flushes
    B. Sleep disturbance
    C. Increased sexual satisfaction
    D. Menorrhagia
    E. Anxiety

28. The long-term consequences of menopause include:
    A. Secondary osteoporosis due to hyperparathyroidism
    B. Increased risk of stroke
    C. Urogenital hypertrophy
    D. Dementia
    E. Increased risk of cardiovascular disease

29. The dual energy X-ray absorptiometry (DEXA) scan:
    A. Is a special X-ray that measures bone mineral density
    B. Is used to diagnose bone fractures
    C. Can help to detect osteopenia
    D. Is safe to be performed during pregnancy
    E. Uses lower levels of radiation than standard X-ray (e.g. chest X-ray)

30. The causes of premature menopause include:
    A. Early menarche
    B. Chromosomal abnormalities
    C. Unilateral oophorectomy
    D. Radiation therapy
    E. Galactosaemia

31. With regard to endometrial pathology and investigation:
    A. Fluid in endometrial cavity on ultrasound scan in postmenopausal women is considered a normal finding.
    B. Hysteroscopy is 100% accurate and detects all endometrial pathology in symptomatic women.
    C. Endometrial cancer is associated with 90% of the cases of postmenopausal bleeding (PMB).
    D. Most endometrial polyps are benign.
    E. Endometrial curettage is 100% accurate in detecting endometrial pathology in symptomatic women.

32. Measurement of the following hormones on day 21 of the menstrual cycle will determine whether the woman had ovulation:
    A. Serum FSH
    B. Urinary FSH
    C. Serum LH
    D. Serum Inhibin B
    E. Progesterone

33. A 60-year-old postmenopausal woman is referred to the rapid-access gynaecological oncology clinic. She is asymptomatic and her ultrasound shows an incidental finding of unilateral unilocular mobile cyst that measures 6 cm.
    A. She would definitely need MRI scan to differentiate benign from malignant cyst.
    B. Laparoscopic oophorectomy is a reasonable option for treatment for those with low risk of malignancy.
    C. If the woman opts to be managed conservatively, it is acceptable to perform repeat ultrasound scans and CA-125 every 3–4 months for a year.
    D. Ultrasound-guided aspiration is the recommended treatment for ovarian cysts in postmenopausal women.
    E. If the risk of malignancy index (RMI) is between 25–250 (moderate risk), laparoscopic oophorectomy is an acceptable option in this woman.

34. A 50-year-old woman presents with heavy menstrual bleeding. An ultrasound scan shows thickened endometrium. Hysteroscopy and endometrial biopsy show endometrial hyperplasia.
    A. If the histology shows simple hyperplasia without atypia, the risk of progression to endometrial cancer is significantly high.
    B. If the histology shows complex hyperplasia she should be offered hysterectomy and bilateral salpingo-oophorectomy.
    C. If the histology shows atypical complex hyperplasia, there is a significant chance of coexistent carcinoma in the uterus.
    D. Endometrial hyperplasia with atypia is less likely to progress to endometrial cancer in comparison to endometrial hyperplasia without atypia.
    E. If the woman has simple hyperplasia without atypia, she can be treated with oral progestogens.

12 GYNAECOLOGICAL PROBLEMS – ANSWERS

SBAs

Answer 1: E

HPV is a DNA virus, associated with cervical, vaginal and vulval cancers. The most common oncogenic subtypes are 16, 18, 31 and 33. HPV 16 and 18 together are responsible for up to 75% of cervical cancers. HPV 6 and 11 cause anogenital warts. Prophylactic HPV vaccination was implemented in the UK in 2008 for girls aged 12–13 years. The quadrivalent vaccine, Gardasil, with protection against HPV types 16 and 18 and also types 6 and 11, is now currently used in the UK vaccination programme. Cervarix, a bivalent vaccine covering HPV 16 and 18 was used for the first 3 years of the UK vaccination programme.

Further reading

Fiander A. Prophylactic human papilloma virus vaccination update. *The Obstetrician & Gynaecologist.* 2009; 11:133–135.

Answer 2: D

Cervical screening is a primary screening tool for cervical malignancy. In England all women between the ages of 25 and 64 years are eligible for a cervical screening test every 3 to 5 years and the frequency interval is based on the age group. Practice is different in Scotland and Wales.

Women in England receive first invitation at the age of 25 years, then 3 yearly screening until the age of 49 years and then 5 yearly from the ages of 50 to 64 years. At or after 65 years, screening is recommended to only those women who have never had screening or had recent abnormal results.

Women who have never been sexually active or have been in a same sex relationship are recommended to have cervical screening, as they are still at risk, despite it being low. Liquid-based cytology is cost effective, easy to prepare and has reduced the rate of inadequate smears significantly.

Further reading

NHSCSP Publication No. 20. *Colposcopy and Programme Management. Guidelines for the NHS Cervical Screening Programme.* 2nd ed. 2010. Available at: www.bsccp.org.uk/colposcopy-resources/colposcopy-and-programme-management-1

Answer 3: C

Bladder wall injection with botulinum toxin A is an invasive procedure offered to women with proven detrusor overactivity that has not responded to conservative management and drug therapy, after MDT review as well as discussing the risks and benefits with women with overactive bladder.

Further reading

NICE clinical guideline 171. *The management of urinary incontinence in women.* 2013. Available at: www.nice.org.uk/nicemedia/live/14271/65143/65143.pdf

Answer 4: D

Therapeutic stimulation in the form of electrical stimulation along with pelvic floor muscle training should not be used routinely.

Further reading

NICE clinical guideline 171. *The management of urinary incontinence in women.* 2013. Available at: www.nice.org.uk/nicemedia/live/14271/65143/65143.pdf

Answer 5: A

Turner's syndrome has the karyotype 45XO. The usual presentation is primary amenorrhoea due to failure of ovarian development. The physical characteristics in Turner's syndrome include short stature, webbed neck and poorly developed secondary sexual characteristics but female genital phenotype. Cardiac abnormalities such as coarctation of aorta are common.

Rarely the karyotype is a combination of 45XO/46XX or 45XO/46XY and is known as Turner's mosaic. In such cases the woman has periods and may be able to conceive and have children.

Further reading

Collins S, Arulkumaran S, et al. *Oxford Handbook of Obstetrics & Gynaecology.* 3rd ed. Oxford: Oxford University Press; 2013.

Answer 6: E

Cervical cytology is a screening test to detect pre-invasive conditions of the cervix. The UK has a good cervical screening programme with appropriate pathways in place for managing abnormal cervical cytology. Screening is offered to women between 25 and 65 years of age. Women less than 25 years of age are not screened as changes (mostly low-grade changes) in the cervix are common in this age group and they mostly resolve by themselves. Changes that do not require any treatment, if detected on smear test would lead to unnecessary treatment and increase workload significantly.

Smears are generally classified as:

- Borderline smear in squamous or glandular cells
- Mild dyskaryosis
- Moderate dyskaryosis
- Severe dyskaryosis
- Glandular neoplasia
- Suspicion of invasive cancer

Although negative smears are generally reassuring, they do not provide 100% protection from cervical cancer, for the following possible reasons:

- The sensitivity of the cervical cytology is 70%.
- The incidence of false negative smears is around 10%.
- Sampling or slide preparation errors plus inaccurate reporting.

In general, the cervical screening programme has worked really well in UK, resulting in a reduction (20%) in the incidence of invasive squamous cervical cancer in the last 28 years and also reduced mortality related to it (7% reduction of cervical cancer every year). HPV testing has been introduced as a triage for low-grade abnormalities (borderline and mild abnormalities) and may be introduced in due course for routine screening.

Further reading

Guidelines for the NHS Cervical Screening Programme. 2nd ed. *Colposcopy and Programme Management.* NHSCSP Publication No. 20. 2010.

Answer 7: C

Cervical cytology is used as screening test to detect pre-invasive conditions of the cervix. Once detected, there are pathways for their follow up and treatment. CIN 1 (low-grade abnormality with low malignant potential) if left untreated will eventually resolve in 50% of the cases; however, if it is persistent, or in cases where the patient is not compliant with follow up, it needs to be treated as the risk of progression to cancer is 1%. CIN 2 and 3 (high-grade abnormalities with a higher malignant potential) have a higher risk of progression to invasive cancer than CIN 1. The risk of progression is 5% and >12% for CIN 2 and CIN 3 respectively.

Further reading

Guidelines for the NHS Cervical Screening Programme. 2nd ed. *Colposcopy and Programme Management.* NHSCSP Publication No. 20. 2010.

Answer 8: E

Cervical cytology is mainly designed to identify squamous abnormalities of the cervix. Rarely (incidence is 1 in 2000 smears) can it pick up a glandular abnormality and this is known as CGIN. It is a preinvasive glandular lesion of the cervix and usually occurs in the older age group.

CGIN is associated with CIN in 50% of cases and an underlying malignancy (adenocarcinoma) in 40% of the cases. Therefore, this abnormality warrants urgent colposcopy referral. These patients should be reviewed in the colposcopy clinic within 2 weeks of referral.

Once seen in the colposcopy clinic, the following approach should be adopted:

- Excisional treatment (LLETZ or cone)
- The depth of cone should be at least 20–25 mm depending on the size of cervix
- Pelvic examination and TVS scan if colposcopy is negative
- +/– Hysteroscopy and biopsy (endometrial biopsy is essential in older women and in those with atypical endometrial cells reported in cervical cytology)
- Ideally follow up after treatment should be lifetime or at least 10 years; the guidelines are changing with the introduction of HPV testing

The preceding approach is important due to the following reasons:

- There are no specific colposcopic features for its diagnosis.
- CGIN is associated with skip lesions higher up in the cervical canal.
- Glandular abnormalities on a cervical smear can be associated with endometrial cancer, fallopian tube cancer or ovarian cancer.

Further reading

Guidelines for the NHS Cervical Screening Programme. 2nd ed. *Colposcopy and Programme Management.* NHSCSP Publication No. 20. 2010.

Answer 9: C

VIN is a preinvasive disease of the vulva. About 5–10% of VIN progresses to vulval cancer. In two-thirds of cases vulval cancer is associated with lichen sclerosus (LS) and in one third of cases it is associated with VIN. It can also be associated with vaginal and cervical intraepithelial neoplasia (field phenomenon).

There are two types of VIN: one that is HPV related, and differentiated VIN, which is secondary to an underlying skin condition namely LS.

Further reading

McCluggage WG. Premalignant lesions of the lower female genital tract: cervix, vagina and vulva. *Pathology.* 2013; 45(3):214–228.

Answer 10: C

Tamoxifen acts as an oestrogen antagonist on breast tissue. Therefore, it is used in the treatment of oestrogen receptor-positive breast cancer in premenopausal women. It is also used in postmenopausal women, although aromatase inhibitors are more frequently used. Its use reduces almost 50% risk of recurrence of breast cancer. It is generally used for 5 years and there is no evidence to recommend its use after 5 years. It acts as an oestrogen agonist on endometrial tissue and therefore can cause endometrial oedema, polyps, endometrial hyperplasia and endometrial cancer. Tamoxifen can be used for ovulation induction in women who are sensitive to clomiphene.

Further reading

Sugerman DT. JAMA patient page: Tamoxifen update. *JAMA*. 2013. 28; 310(8):866.

Answer 11: B

Tumour Markers and Cancer

Oncofetal Proteins	Cancer
CEA	Colon and pancreatic cancer
AFP	Hepatocellular, germ cell tumour, yolk sac tumour, non-seminomatous germ cell tumour and embryonal carcinoma
Hormones	Cancer
Catecholamines and VMA	Pheochromocytoma
Calcitonin	Medullary carcinoma of thyroid
Beta human chorionic gonadotrophin (βhCG)	Gestational trophoblastic tumour, Choriocarcinoma
Enzymes and proteins	Cancer
CA 15.3	Breast cancer
CA 19.9	Upper GI and pancreatic cancer
CA-125	Epithelial ovarian cancer and primary peritoneal cancer
PSA and PAP	Prostatic cancer
Immunoglobulins	Multiple myeloma

Further reading

Collins S, Arulkumaran S, et al. *Oxford Handbook of Obstetrics & Gynaecology*. 3rd ed. Oxford: Oxford University Press; 2013.

EMQs

Answers 1–3

1. G
Involuntary loss of urine caused when the bladder pressure exceeds the urethral pressure is known as stress incontinence. These symptoms generally occur due to weakness of the pelvic floor muscles.

2. J
The most common cause of urinary symptoms following delivery is urinary tract infection. A mid-stream urine sample for culture and sensitivity should be sent for diagnosis and the woman treated with the appropriate antibiotics.

3. B
Detrusor contractions during the bladder-filling phase cause the bladder pressure to exceed the urethral pressure, leading to incontinence. This is called detrusor instability or overactive bladder.

Further reading

NICE clinical guideline No. 171. *The management of urinary incontinence in women.*
   Available at: guidance.nice.org.uk/CG171

Answers 4–6

4. A
The options to be considered here are total abdominal hysterectomy or total abdominal hysterectomy with bilateral salpingo-oophorectomy (BSO). Symptoms of menopause and long-term effects along with the pros and cons of HRT should be considered with BSO. Myomectomy is not suitable treatment as she is 47 years old and has completed her family.

5. D
Vaginal hysterectomy is the most appropriate surgical option in this case due to prolapse and menorrhagia not amenable to medical treatment.

6. C
For women with postmenopausal bleeding and endometrial thickness of >4 mm, hysteroscopy and endometrial biopsy should be performed to rule out endometrial pathology.

Further reading

SIGN Guideline 61. *Investigation of post-menopausal bleeding.* 2002. Available at:
   www.sign.ac.uk/guidelines/fulltext/61/section4.html

Answers 7–9

7. B

Laparoscopy and dye test should be offered for women with comorbidities such as pelvic inflammatory disease, previous ectopic or endometriosis, so that tubal and pelvic pathology can be assessed at the same time. For women with no comorbidities HSG should be offered to screen for tubal occlusion as it is reliable, less invasive and cost effective. Hysterosalpingo-contrast-ultrasonography is an alternative to HSG where expertise is available.

Further reading

NICE clinical guideline 156. *Fertility*. 2013. Available at: www.nice.org.uk/ nicemedia/live/14078/62769/62769.pdf

8. J

Semen analysis results show mild oligozoospermia with a sperm concentration of <15 million/ml and hence the test should be repeated 3 months after the initial test to allow time for the cycle of spermatozoa formation to be completed. However, if there is azoospermia or severe oligozoospermia a repeat test should be done as soon as possible.

Further reading

NICE clinical guideline 156. *Fertility*. 2013. Available at: www.nice.org.uk/ nicemedia/live/14078/62769/62769.pdf

9. C

In women with irregular prolonged menstrual cycles serum progesterone should be done later in the cycle – as, in this case, on day 28 of a 35 days cycle – and repeated weekly until the next menstrual cycle starts.

Further reading

NICE clinical guideline 156. *Fertility*. 2013. Available at: www.nice.org.uk/ nicemedia/live/14078/62769/62769.pdf

Answers 10–12

10. H

Urinary retention with overflow incontinence is a typical presentation in the postnatal period. Prolonged labour, regional anaesthesia, forceps delivery and perineal trauma predispose to urinary retention. Small voiding volumes should be of concern. Bladder scan to check post-void residual and ensure complete bladder emptying should be performed.

11. J

Urodynamic stress incontinence is the involuntary leakage of urine during increased intra-abdominal pressure in the absence of detrusor contractions and can only be diagnosed by urodynamic studies. Stress urinary incontinence is a symptom/complaint of involuntary leakage of urine on effort or exertion, or on sneezing or coughing.

12. F
Overactive bladder is a chronic condition, defined as urgency with or without urge incontinence, usually with frequency or nocturia. Detrusor overactivity is probably the underlying condition, but the diagnosis can be confirmed on urodynamic testing.

Further reading

NICE clinical guideline 171. *The management of urinary incontinence in women.* Available at: guidance.nice.org.uk/CG171

Collins S, Arulkumaran S, et al. *Oxford Handbook of Obstetrics & Gynaecology.* 3rd ed. Oxford: Oxford University Press; 2013.

Answers 13–15

13. A
Supervised pelvic floor muscle training of at least 3 months duration should be offered as a first-line treatment to women with stress or mixed urinary incontinence (NICE).

14. H
For women with urge or mixed incontinence, bladder training for a minimum of 6 weeks should be offered as a first-line treatment (NICE).

15. G
The surgical options for women with urodynamic stress incontinence, where the conservative management is not successful, include insertion of a synthetic mid-urethral tape, colposuspension or autologous rectal fascial sling procedures (NICE).

Further reading

NICE clinical guideline 171. *The management of urinary incontinence in women.* 2013. Available at: www.nice.org.uk/nicemedia/live/14271/65143/65143.pdf

Answers 16–18

16. C
In women with abdominal pains in early pregnancy and localized tenderness, the diagnosis of ectopic pregnancy should be considered until proven otherwise.

17. F
The history, symptoms and signs are suggestive of an acute infection of the lower genital tract: pelvic inflammatory disease.

18. B

The likely diagnosis is ovarian cyst accident: torsion or rupture, given the clinical scenario of acute onset of pains in presence of an intrauterine pregnancy and an ovarian cyst.

Further reading

Collins S, Arulkumaran S, et al. *Oxford Handbook of Obstetrics & Gynaecology*. 3rd ed. Oxford: Oxford University Press; 2013.

Answers 19–21

19. B
20. J
21. H

- Lactate dehydrogenase (LDH), α-FP and hCG should be measured in all women under age 40 years with a complex ovarian mass because of the possibility of germ cell tumours.
- The generally accepted definition of an ovarian cyst is: 'a fluid-containing structure more than 30 mm in diameter'.
- Women with simple cystic structures less than 50 mm in diameter do not generally require follow-up as these cysts are likely to be physiological and almost always resolve within 3 menstrual cycles.
- Asymptomatic women with simple cysts of 30–50 mm in diameter do not require follow-up, cysts 50–70 mm require yearly ultrasound follow-up and cysts more than 70 mm in diameter should be considered for either further imaging (MRI) or surgical intervention due to difficulties in examining the entire cyst adequately at time of ultrasound.
- The recurrence of endometriomas and their symptoms are reduced by excisional surgery, more so than by drainage and ablation. Subsequent spontaneous pregnancy rates in women who were previously sub-fertile are also improved with this treatment.

Further reading

RCOG Green-top guideline No. 62. *Management of suspected ovarian masses in premenopausal women*. 2011. Available at: www.rcog.org.uk/womens-health/clinical-guidance/ovarian-masses-premenopausal-women-management-suspected-green-top-62

RCOG Green-top guideline No. 24. *The investigation and management of endometriosis*. 2006. Available at: www.rcog.org.uk/womens-health/clinical-guidance/investigation-and-management-endometriosis-green-top-24

Answers 22–24

22. I
23. D
24. A

- Simple, unilateral, unilocular ovarian cysts, less than 5 cm in diameter, have a low risk of malignancy. It is recommended that, in the presence of normal serum CA-125 levels, they can be managed conservatively unless symptomatic.
- Aspiration is not recommended for the management of ovarian cysts in postmenopausal women.
- Laparoscopic management of ovarian cysts in postmenopausal women should involve oophorectomy (usually bilateral) rather than cystectomy.
- All ovarian cysts that are suspicious of malignancy in a postmenopausal woman, as indicated by a high risk of malignancy index, clinical suspicion or findings at laparoscopy, are likely to require a full staging laparotomy by the gynaecological oncology team in a cancer centre, through an extended midline incision. This procedure should include:
  - Cytology: ascites or washings
  - Laparotomy with clear documentation
  - Biopsies from adhesions and suspicious areas
  - Total abdominal hysterectomy, bilateral salpingo-oophorectomy and infra-colic omentectomy

- CA-125 blood serum level and urgent pelvic ultrasound should be carried out in women with the following symptoms:
  - Persistent abdominal distension
  - Feeling abdominal fullness
  - Loss of appetite
  - Pelvic or abdominal pain

- Increased urinary urgency and/or frequency (particularly if occurring more than 12 times per month and especially if she is over 50 years)

Further reading

RCOG Green-top guideline No. 34. *Ovarian cysts in postmenopausal women*. 2010. Available at: www.rcog.org.uk/womens-health/clinical-guidance/ovarian-cysts-postmenopausal-women-green-top-34

SIGN 135. *Management of epithelial ovarian cancer*. 2013. Available at: www.sign.ac.uk/pdf/sign135.pdf

Answers 25–27

25. F
26. G
27. H

- Up to 33% of *in vitro* fertilization (IVF) cycles have mild ovarian hyperstimulation syndrome (OHSS) and 3–8% are complicated by moderate or severe OHSS.
- Women with mild OHSS and many with moderate OHSS can be managed on an outpatient basis.
- Analgesia using paracetamol or codeine is appropriate. Nonsteroidal anti-inflammatory drugs should not be used.
- Treatment for pain symptoms presumed to be caused by endometriosis includes counselling, adequate analgesia, progestogens or the combined oral contraceptive. It is unclear whether combined oral contraceptives should be taken conventionally, continuously or in a tricycle regimen (i.e. 3 packets back-to-back). A gonadotrophin-releasing hormone (GnRH) agonist may be taken but this class of drug is more expensive and associated with more adverse effects and concerns about bone density.
- Laparoscopic ovarian cystectomy is recommended if an ovarian endometrioma is ≥4 cm in diameter in order to:
  - confirm the diagnosis histologically;
  - reduce the risk of infection;
  - improve access to follicles;
  - improve ovarian response; and
  - prevent endometriosis progression.

- The woman should be counselled regarding the risks of reduced ovarian function after surgery and the loss of the ovary.

Further reading

RCOG Green-top guideline No. 5. *The management of ovarian hyperstimulation syndrome*. 2006. Available at: www.rcog.org.uk/womens-health/clinical-guidance /management-ovarian-hyperstimulation-syndrome-green-top-5

MCQs

1A: False – COCPs have not shown to be of benefit in relieving PMS symptoms. It is proposed that mineralocorticoid activity of the progestogen (in second-generation pills) may regenerate PMS symptoms. In contrast, Yasmin contains drosperinone, which has anti-mineralocorticoid and anti-androgenic progestogen and helps in the relief of some of the symptoms of PMS. There is no evidence to support continuous rather than cyclical use of COCP.

1B: False – Cognitive behavioural therapy should be offered to everybody and could be extremely effective, even in severe cases.

1C: False – There is no evidence to support continuous rather than cyclical use of COCP.

1D: False – SSRIs can be used either continuously or only in the luteal phase and have been shown to be effective in improving both physical and psychological PMS symptoms.

1E: True – The evidence for use of complementary therapy is limited. It is considered appropriate to try those therapies that have not been shown to be detrimental in view of poor understanding of the aetiology of premenstrual syndrome.

Further reading

RCOG Green-top guideline No. 48. *Management of premenstrual syndrome.* 2007. Available at: www.rcog.org.uk/womens-health/clinical-guidance/management-premenstrual-syndrome-green-top-48

2A: True – Unopposed use of oestrogen has been shown to significantly increase the risk of endometrial cancer.

2B: False
2C: False
2D: False
2E: False

HRT increases the risk of:

- ovarian cancer (there is slight increase in the risk of ovarian cancer in women taking oestrogen-only HRT but the risk with combined HRT is unknown);
- breast cancer (especially when oestrogen preparations are used); and
- thromboembolic disease.

Further reading

Collins S, Arulkumaran S, et al. *Oxford Handbook of Obstetrics & Gynaecology.* 3rd ed. Oxford: Oxford University Press; 2013.

3A: False
3B: True
3C: True
3D: True
3E: False

Bacterial vaginosis (BV) is a polymicrobial infection of the vagina. It is caused by an overgrowth of anaerobes and most women present with vaginal discharge. *Gardnerella vaginalis*, also known as *Haemophilus vaginalis*, is a facultative anaerobic, non-flagellated, non-spore forming bacteria. It is recognized as one of the organisms responsible for causing bacterial vaginosis. The other organisms involved in this pathology include bacteriods, pepto-streptococcus, fuso-bacterium, mycoplasma hominis, mobilucus and veilonella.

Women typically present with a thin grey homogenous vaginal discharge that has a characteristic fishy odour (alkalinity of semen may cause a release of volatile amines from the vaginal discharge – forms the basis for a whiff test). The fishy smell is mainly recognized after sexual intercourse. Vulval itching, dysuria and dyspareunia are rare, unlike with *Trichomonas vaginalis* infection. It is also known to cause vault infection following hysterectomy and also pelvic infection after abortion. In pregnant women it has been associated with premature rupture of membranes and preterm delivery. The following are recognized as risk factors for the development of BV: vaginal douching, prolonged antibiotic use, decrease in oestrogen production, presence of intrauterine device (especially copper IUD) and increase in number of sexual partners.

There is an increase in vaginal PH (>4.5) as it is associated with a decrease in lactobacilli (responsible for maintaining the acidic pH) in the vagina (normally this acidic pH prevents the overgrowth of other organisms in the vagina). Wet-mount saline preparation with vaginal discharge shows 'clue' cells (vaginal epithelial cells have a stippled appearance due to adherence of cocobacilli) under low- and high-power microscopy. The drug used for treatment is metronidazole. Its use should be avoided during the first trimester. Topical clindamycin and metronidazole are also useful in bringing the vaginal flora to normal.

Amsel's criteria for the diagnosis of bacterial vaginosis are:

- thin white homogenous discharge;
- increase in vaginal pH (>4.5);
- clue cells on microscopy; and
- whiff test or KOH test: when a few drops of alkali (10% KOH) are added to vaginal secretions, a fishy smell is released.

At least three of the four should be present to make the diagnosis.

Further reading

Collins S, Arulkumaran S, et al. *Oxford Handbook of Obstetrics & Gynaecology*. 3rd ed. Oxford: Oxford University Press; 2013.

4A: True – HPV 1, 2 and 4 are not sexually transmitted.
4B: True – These women are usually asymptomatic and the HPV infection is transient and resolves by itself.
4C: False
4D: True
4E: False – The persistence of HPV infection in the cervix leads to the development of CIN and subsequently to cervical cancer.

HPV is a double-stranded DNA virus. It has a predilection for the transformation zone on the cervix. It causes preinvasive changes in the surface squamous epithelium, which is known as CIN. CIN is classified as grade 1–3 depending on the depth from the basement membrane that is affected. HPV with CIN 1 are classified as low-grade lesions while CIN 2-3 are classed as high-grade lesions.

HPV infection can be sexually transmitted (can be acquired from having sex with an infected person at any age) and is more common in women under 25 years of age. These women are usually asymptomatic and the infection is often transient. However, if the HPV persists in the cervix, it may lead to high-grade CIN lesions and ultimately cervical cancer. Almost all cervical cancers are caused by HPV infections. In the UK, HPV 16 accounts for 60–80% of high-grade CIN lesions and cervical cancer. The remainder are mostly caused by HPV types 18, 31, 33 and 35. HPV 6 and 11 (low-risk types) cause genital warts that are generally benign. The other high-risk HPV types include 39, 45, 51, 52, 56 and 58, which have also been associated with cervical cancer. Palmar and plantar warts are not sexually transmitted and are caused by HPV 1, 2 and 4. Recently, HPV infections have been found to cause oropharyngeal cancers, which are linked to HPV 16.

The main risk factors for genital HPV include:

- Starting sexual activity at early age (16 years or younger) when the transformation zone is maturing
- Multiple sexual partners
- Women younger than 25 years of age
- Having a male partner who is uncircumcised
- Immunosuppression (e.g. women on immunosuppressive therapy following kidney transplant or women with HIV)

The best way to prevent HPV infection is to avoid contact (skin to skin, which can be oral, anal or genital). A monogamous relationship with an uninfected partner is the best strategy to prevent HPV infection; however, it is difficult to know who is infected and who is not because most HPV infections are asymptomatic. The use of condoms can decrease the transmission of HPV infection but uncovered areas can still be infected. Therefore, condoms are not known to completely protect against HPV virus infection.

Further reading

Collins S, Arulkumaran S, et al. *Oxford Handbook of Obstetrics & Gynaecology*. 3rd ed. Oxford: Oxford University Press; 2013.

5A: True – Adenomyosis is the presence of endometrial tissue within the myometrium. It can be associated with endometriosis in pelvis. It is an oestrogen-dependent condition and its prevalence decreases after the menopause, as the oestrogen levels fall. The woman usually presents with menorrhagia and dysmenorrhoea (uterine tenderness may be present during periods). Treatment options include Mirena IUS in young women and hysterectomy in older women. **5B: False** – Small subserous fibroids usually do not cause any menstrual symptoms but can cause pressure symptoms (e.g. constipation, heaviness in the pelvis and bladder symptoms). Submucous and intramural fibroids can cause both menorrhagia and dysmenorrhoea, especially if the endometrial lining is distorted.

5C: True – Women with endometriosis usually present with dyspareunia, dysmenorrhoea and dyschezia.

5D: False – Women with endometrial atrophy can present with postmenopausal bleeding.

5E: False – Mirena IUS is the first-line treatment for women presenting with menorrhagia due to dysfunctional uterine bleeding (DUB).

Further reading

Collins S, Arulkumaran S, et al. *Oxford Handbook of Obstetrics & Gynaecology*. 3rd ed. Oxford: Oxford University Press; 2013.

6A: True
6B: True
6C: False
6D: False
6E: False

Secondary amenorrhoea is defined as the absence of a menstrual period for 6 months in a woman who has regular menstrual periods, or the absence of a menstrual period equivalent to three previous cycle lengths.

Causes of secondary amenorrhoea

- Hypothalamic causes
    - Excessive weight loss (or sudden weight loss)
    - Excessive exercise
    - Eating disorders e.g. anorexia nervosa (weight loss more than 25% of body weight)

- Hormonal
    - Hyperprolactinaemia
    - PCOS
    - Obesity
    - Premature ovarian failure
    - Hypopituitarism
    - Hypogonadotrophic hypogonadism
    - Thyroid dysfunction
    - Cushing disease

- Ovarian causes
    - Premature ovarian failure (POF): this is defined as the onset of menopause before the age of 40 years (incidence: 1%). It is mainly caused by failure of ovaries to produce oestrogens. In most cases it is associated with another auto-immune disease such as Addison disease, thyroid disease and hypoparathyroidism. The other causes of POF include galactosaemia, chemotherapy, radiotherapy, hysterectomy and bilateral salpingo-oophorectomy.
    - PCOS

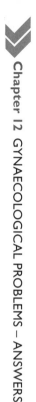

- Pituitary causes
  - Damage caused by radiotherapy, head injury, tuberculosis and sarcoidosis
  - Sheehan syndrome: necrosis of the pituitary gland resulting from severe hypotension during pregnancy and delivery e.g. massive PPH. This leads to releasing hormone deficiency (e.g. ACTH and TSH).
  - Prolactin-secreting pituitary adenoma

- Outflow tract problems
  - Asherman's syndrome: intrauterine adhesions typically related to postpartum endometrial curettage or post-miscarriage or post-termination of pregnancy
  - Cervical stenosis

- Chronic illnesses
  - Tuberculosis
  - Chronic renal disease

- Malignancy

Further reading

Collins S, Arulkumaran S, et al. *Oxford Handbook of Obstetrics & Gynaecology.* 3rd ed. Oxford: Oxford University Press; 2013.

7A: False
7B: False
7C: True
7D: True
7E: True

CA-125 can be used for screening of high-risk women (e.g. BRCA1 and BRCA2 positive or family history of breast/ovarian cancer or personal history of ovarian cancer), particularly when they are still waiting to complete their family and do not wish to have a prophylactic oophorectomy. It can also be used to assess disease status (ovarian cancer) and response to therapy (to check CA-125 levels following chemotherapy and surgery). However, CA-125 is a glycoprotein produced by most (80%) of advanced epithelial ovarian cancer but only by 50% of stage I ovarian disease. CA-125 lacks specificity and can be raised in benign conditions of the pelvis, which include fibroids, pelvic inflammatory disease, endometriosis, diverticulitis and inflammatory bowel disease. In view of this CA-125 is not used as a screening test in the general population.

CA-125 is used with ultrasound findings (solid, multicystic, bilateral, ascites, irregular) and the menopausal status to calculate the risk of malignancy index (RMI) in order to plan the type of management (surgery or conservative by follow up ultrasound scan), urgency of management and decision to refer to a cancer centre.

RMI is calculated by multiplying the following three parameters:

1. USG features (U = 0 for USG score of 0, U = 1 for USG score of 1 and U = 3 for USG score of 2–5). A score of 1 is given to each of the following features seen on USG: solid, multicystic, bilateral, ascites, irregular.

2. Menopausal status (use 3 for postmenopausal women and 1 for premenopausal women)
3. CA-125 levels (actual value from the blood test)

The final number acquired after multiplication of the above factors is regarded as RMI. This number determines the risk of ovarian cancer e.g. <25 is considered low risk and the risk of cancer is <3%, RMI 25–250 is considered moderate risk and the risk of cancer is 20%, and RMI >250 is considered high risk for malignancy and the risk of cancer is 75%. If RMI is >250, the woman would need to be referred to the cancer centre.

Further reading

RCOG Green-top guideline No. 34. *Ovarian cysts in postmenopausal women.* 2003. Available at: www.rcog.org.uk/womens-health/clinical-guidance/ovarian-cysts-postmenopausal-women-green-top-34

8A: False
8B: True
8C: True
8D: False
8E: True

Serum testosterone levels are normally <2 nmol/l in women. They can be raised in ovarian or adrenal conditions. Ovarian conditions causing raised serum testosterone levels include theca cell tumours, arrhenoblastoma, gynandroblastoma, Leydig cell tumour (levels >5 nmol/l), ovarian hyperthecosis and polycystic ovarian syndrome (levels >3 nmol/l). Adrenal conditions causing raised serum testosterone levels include Cushing syndrome (levels >4 nmol/l) and adrenal tumours (if levels are >7 nmol/l suspect an androgen secreting tumour).

Further reading

Collins S, Arulkumaran S, et al. *Oxford Handbook of Obstetrics & Gynaecology.* 3rd ed. Oxford: Oxford University Press; 2013.

9A: False
9B: False
9C: False
9D: False
9E: False

Germ cell tumours are common in young women and may produce tumour markers specific to their cell type. These include:

- AFP: endodermal sinus tumour and embryonal carcinoma
- βhCG: non-gestational choriocarcinoma
- βhCG: gestational trophoblastic disease
- βhCG may be raised: dysgerminoma
- Placental alkaline phosphatase and lactate dehydrogenase (LDH): dysgerminoma (especially metastatic disease)

- Granulosa cell tumours: oestrogens and inhibin
- Androgens (testosterone): Sertoli-Leydig cell tumours

The above tumour markers should be measured especially in young women. Knowing the specific tumour markers will aid in diagnosis, treatment (surgery or chemotherapy), to check response to treatment and follow up of patients.

Further reading

Collins S, Arulkumaran S, et al. *Oxford Handbook of Obstetrics & Gynaecology*. 3rd ed. Oxford: Oxford University Press; 2013.

10A: True
10B: True
10C: False
10D: True
10E: False

Hirsutism refers to male pattern distribution of body hair (e.g. beard or hair on the chest) caused by sensitization of the hair follicles by testosterone. Once sensitized the hair continues to grow. This explains the recurrence of the hair growth following stopping of anti-androgen therapy, unless the cause for hirsutism is removed.

The treatment of hirsutism requires treatment of the underlying cause.

1. Lifestyle changes: weight reduction in women with PCOS
2. COCP if not trying to conceive
   - Progestational component: LH suppression and 5-alpha reductase inhibition
   - Oestrogenic component: increases SHBG

3. Medroxyprogesterone acetate if COCP is contraindicated
   - LH suppression
   - SHBG decreases (counterproductive)
   - Testosterone clearance increases (liver enzyme induction)

4. Cosmetic approaches
   - Permanent hair removal by using laser and electrolysis
   - Temporary hair removal by using chemical depilatories, bleaching, waxing, tweezing, mechanical epilators

Further reading

Collins S, Arulkumaran S, et al. *Oxford Handbook of Obstetrics & Gynaecology*. 3rd ed. Oxford: Oxford University Press; 2013.

Bader T. *OB/GYN Secrets*. 3rd ed. Maryland Heights: Mosby; 2004.

11A: True
11B: True
11C: False
11D: False
11E: True

Aetiology of puberty menorrhagia

- Anovulation is the most common cause of puberty menorrhagia. Following menarche it generally takes more than a year to regulate ovulation and their periods. PCOS is also not uncommon at this age.
- Bleeding disorders should be ruled out in young women with intractable menorrhagia. These include Von Willebrand disease; Christmas disease; haemophilia A; factor V, VII, VIII, IX, X and XI deficiency; idiopathic thrombocytopenic purpura; and platelet dysfunction.
- Thyroid dysfunction: hypothyroidism should be excluded. Acquired Von Willebrand disease is associated with hypothyroidism and is seen mainly in women.

Investigations

- Full blood count, platelet count, clotting profile
- Blood film to rule leukaemia
- All the above clotting factors if indicated. VWF: AC assay is the most sensitive assay for screening of Von Willebrand disease. Bleeding time and APTT is prolonged in women with severe haemophilia. Genetic testing can be done for this condition.
- Thyroid function tests as indicated on clinical grounds.

The RCOG guidelines for the management of menorrhagia recommend testing for bleeding disorders only when there are features in history and examination of bleeding disorders. However, the American College of Obstetricians and Gynaecologist (ACOG) guidelines recommend screening for Von Willebrand disease in all adolescents with menorrhagia.

Further reading

Harper A (ed). *Haemorrhage and Thrombosis for the MRCOG and Beyond.* London: RCOG Press; 2005.

12A: False
12B: False
12C: False
12D: True
12E: True

First-line treatment for puberty menorrhagia is medical.
The most commonly used first-line options include:

- Tranexamic acid
- COCP: is commonly used in the treatment of menorrhagia. It causes endometrial atrophy and decreases endometrial prostaglandins and fibrinolysis. Menstrual loss is decreased by 50%. This can be used back-to-back for 3 months to build haemoglobin levels. COCP are especially useful in the presence of an irregular menstrual cycle and the need for contraception.
- Progestogens: anovulatory bleeding is common in this age group. Oral progestogens 5 mg three times daily from day 5 to 26 of the cycle cyclically can be given. This reduces the menstrual blood loss by up to 30%. It can also be used

back-to-back for 3 months to build up the haemoglobin levels. Progestogens are advisable in women with irregular and unpredictable cycle. They are also used as second-line therapy for treatment of inherited bleeding disorder not responding to the other treatments or when these treatments are contraindicated.

- Desmopressin or 1-deamino-8-D-arginine vasopressin (DDAVP) nasal spray is a vasopressin analogue that causes rapid release of factor VIII and VWF from endothelial cells, hence increasing their plasma levels. It is mainly effective in women with type 1 Von Willebrand disease and mild to moderate haemophilia. It is important to give a test dose prior to treatment in order to identify responders from non-responders. It is usually given in the first 2–3 days of menstrual cycle. It is used as intranasal spray or administered by subcutaneous injection in women with Von Willebrand disease.
- Mirena IUS can be considered for long-term management following resolution of acute bleeding.
- The role of danazol and GnRH analogues is not well defined.

Further reading

Harper A (ed). *Haemorrhage and Thrombosis for the MRCOG and Beyond*. London: RCOG Press; 2005.

13A: False
13B: False
13C: False
13D: False
13E: False

DUB is a diagnosis of exclusion. It is defined as regular heavy menstrual bleeding without any postcoital or intermenstrual bleeding or any palpable pelvic pathology and should have a normal cervical smear result. It is mainly due to an imbalance in the hypothalamo-pituitary-ovarian axis.

Investigations should be guided by the history and examination findings.

- Full blood count: she may be anaemic and need iron therapy or a blood transfusion if found to have severe anaemia.
- Cervical smear: if she is not up to date.
- Pregnancy test: if the history is suggestive or if there is any chance that she could be pregnant.
- Thyroid function test and coagulation screen: only indicated if there is a significant history suggestive of these conditions.
- Transvaginal scan: to assess endometrial thickness and exclude uterine fibroids, ovarian masses and uterine polyps.
- Endometrial biopsy: is indicated if there is intermenstrual bleeding, ultrasound scan shows endometrial hyperplasia, polyps, if the woman is over the age of 45 years (to exclude malignancy), or the woman is unresponsive to previous treatment.
- Hysteroscopy and endometrial biopsy: pipelle endometrial biopsy can be performed in the outpatient clinic. However, if pipelle is not possible in the clinic a hysteroscopy and endometrial biopsy should be performed. It is also indicated if the ultrasound scan is suggestive of uterine polyps of submucous fibroids.

Management of DUB and heavy menstrual bleeding (menorrhagia) due to other causes

Medical

- First line

Mirena IUS

- It decreases menstrual blood loss by 90% and has fewer side effects than systemic progestogens. It can also be used as a contraceptive.
- Second line

Antifibrinolytics (i.e. Tranexamic acid)

- Should be taken during menstruation only. Its use for the whole month may increase the risk of thromboembolism, about which the patient should be warned.
- It decreases menstrual blood loss by 50%.

NSAIDs (i.e. mefenamic acid)

- It decreases menstrual blood loss by 30%.
- It can also be effective for women with dysmenorrhoea.
- Side effects are similar to those of aspirin (gastrointestinal).
- It is not to be used in asthmatics.

COCP

- It decreases menstrual blood loss by 40–50%.
- It can also be used as a contraceptive.
- It may have systemic side effects.
- It may have increased risks in older women and those who smoke.
- Third line

Oral progestogens

- It decreases menstrual blood loss by up to 30%.
- Oral progestogens 5 mg can be given three times daily from day 5 to 26 of the cycle cyclically.
- It can be used back-to-back for 3 months to build up the haemoglobin level.
- Progestogens are advisable in women with irregular and unpredictable cycles.

GnRH analogues

- They produce amenorrhoea and therefore decrease menstrual blood loss by almost 100%.
- Their use is limited to 3–6 months because of the ensuing medical menopause and its sequelae (osteoporosis, hot flushes and night sweats).
- It is used as a short-term treatment while awaiting surgery.
- It is also used for women with fibroids prior to surgery.

Surgical treatment
Hysteroscopy

- It is used to remove polyps or submucous fibroids.

Endometrial ablation

- Mostly used in older women who have completed their family.
- Not suitable for young women who wish to have more children.
- Traditionally transcervical resection of endometrium (TCRE) was used but, with newer and safer techniques, this is no longer used.
- Now more likely to be microwave probe or thermal balloon ablation.
- Risks include uterine perforation, infection and subfertility.
- Menstrual loss might remain unacceptable and might require further surgery (10-40% would need repeat surgery at 5 years).
- The woman's expectations might not be met (e.g. dysmenorrhoea and premenstrual syndrome might not be relieved).
- Subsequent pregnancy is contraindicated.

Transcervical resection of fibroids (TCRF)

- Used mainly to resect submucous fibroids.
- Suitable for fibroids <4 cm.
- Risks include bleeding, infection, uterine perforation, fluid overload and hyponatraemia, and cerebral oedema due to fluid overload. Rarely, thermal bowel and bladder injury may occur.

Myomectomy

- Suitable for large intramural fibroids with menorrhagia.
- Also used if submucous fibroids are larger than 4 cm.
- Can be performed either by laparoscopy or by open laparotomy.
- GnRH analogues can be used to decrease fibroid diameter prior to surgery.

Hysterectomy

- Involves removal of the uterus to treat menorrhagia.
- The last line of treatment unless the patient declines other forms of treatment.
- Not first-line treatment for young women.
- Mainly used for perimenopausal women with menorrhagia.
- 100% cure and 90% satisfaction but 3% risk of life-threatening complications.

Further reading

Collins S, Arulkumaran S, et al. *Oxford Handbook of Obstetrics & Gynaecology*. 3rd ed. Oxford: Oxford University Press; 2013.

14A: True
14B: False
14C: False
14D: True
14E: True

- Hirsutism: excessive growth of body hair in anatomic sites where growth is considered to be a male-pattern distribution (normal pattern of hair distribution is age and race dependent)
- Incidence: 10% in developed countries

Pathophysiology of Hirsutism

Increased Exposure to Androgen		Increased end-Organ Sensitivity	
Exogenous androgens	Androgens Progestogens with androgenic potential	5-alpha reductase activity in the skin	Insulin growth factor-1 in patients with insulin resistance and hyperinsulinaemia
Increased production	Tumours Enzyme defects Cushing syndrome Hyperinsulinaemia Increased LH levels stimulate the CA cells		
Alterations in binding globulins (SHBG)	Hyperinsulinaemia Liver disease Androgens Hyperprolactnemia Hypothyroidism		

Aetiology of Hirsutism

Ovary	Adrenal gland	External causes
PCOS 95% Androgen-secreting Tumours <1% Luteoma of pregnancy<1%	Congenital adrenal hyperplasia <1% Cushing syndrome <1% Androgen-secreting Tumours <1%	Iatrogenic hirsutism <1% Drugs with androgenic effect (anabolic steroids, danazol, testosterone) <1%

Further reading

Collins S, Arulkumaran S, et al. *Oxford Handbook of Obstetrics & Gynaecology*. 3rd ed. Oxford: Oxford University Press; 2013.

Bader T. *OB/GYN Secrets*. 3rd ed. Maryland Heights: Mosby; 2004.

15A: False – Drug history is very important.
15B: True
15C: True
15D: True
15E: True

History of hirsutism should include:

- Age of onset: adults present with late-onset congenital adrenal hyperplasia.
- Rate of onset (within months): rapid onset indicates androgen producing ovarian and adrenal gland tumours. This is usually associated with signs of virilization. Slow onset can be due to either PCOS, constitutional or drugs.
- Pregnancy: luteoma is a known cause of hirsutism in pregnancy.
- Menstrual cycle: irregularity of menstrual cycle, oligomenorrhoea and amenorrhoea are all common in women with PCOS.
- Associated symptoms: voice changes, increased muscular mass, male distribution of hair and clitoromegaly (signs of virilization) are mainly present when the serum androgen levels are very high. These signs are seen in women with androgen-producing ovarian (Sertoli–Leydig cell tumours or arrhenoblastoma) or adrenal tumours (adrenal adenoma).
- Drug history: Danazol, anabolic steroids and progestogens with androgenic action (Minoxidil causes hypertrichosis).
- Genetic factors: PCOS, type 2 diabetes, increased sensitivity to 5-alpha reductase.
- Endocrinology: Cushing syndrome, acromegaly.

Further reading

Collins S, Arulkumaran S, et al. *Oxford Handbook of Obstetrics & Gynaecology*. 3rd ed. Oxford: Oxford University Press; 2013.

Bader T. *OB/GYN Secrets*. 3rd ed. Maryland Heights: Mosby; 2004.

16A: False
16B: False – Extremely high levels of 17-OH progesterone are seen in women with late-onset congenital adrenal hyperplasia.
16C: True
16D: True
16E: True

- History: onset, duration, drug, familial and hormonal disorders
- Examination
  - Look for pattern of hair distribution
  - Exclude hypertrichosis (localized overgrowth of hair)
  - Look for signs of virilization (increase in muscle mass, voice changes to male type and clitoromegaly)
  - Use Ferriman–Gallwey scoring system to grade hirsutism. It is graded as grade 1 (minimal hirsutism) – grade 4 (frank virilization).
    - Normal: score of <8
    - Mild hirsutism: score of 8–15
    - Moderate to severe hirsutism: score of >15

- Acanthosis nigricans (a sign of hyperinsulinaemia and insulin resistance)
- Look for any signs of Cushing syndrome (facies, buffalo hump, striae on the body and increased blood pressure (BP))
- Look for any signs of acromegaly (gigantism)
- Investigations
  - Testosterone levels: is produced both in adrenal gland and ovary
  - DHEAS: almost exclusively produced in the adrenal gland
  - Oral glucose tolerance test (OGTT) → Insulin resistance. It is seen in PCOS.
  - 17-hydroxyprogesterone → rule out CAH
  - 24-hour urinary cortisol levels, early morning serum cortisol before 9 am and dexamethasone suppression test
- Transvaginal scan (TVS) to rule out any ovarian pathology (PCOS or ovarian tumours)

Further reading

Collins S, Arulkumaran, S, et al. Oxford Handbook of Obstetrics & Gynaecology. 3rd ed. Oxford: Oxford University Press; 2013.

17A: True
17B: True
17C: False – Ketoconazole is used in the treatment of hirsutism.
17D: True
17E: False – Haloperidol is an anti-psychotic drug.

The treatment of hirsutism depends on the underlying cause.

- PCOS
  - Lifestyle changes: weight reduction
  - COCP if the woman is not trying to conceive. It will also help to regularize periods and can provide contraception. The progestational component of COCP causes LH suppression and inhibits 5-alpha reductase enzyme. The oestrogen component increases SHBG levels. Therefore, both together reduces the luteinizing hormone (LH) stimulation of theca cells in the ovary and reduces the free serum androgen or testosterone levels.
- Medroxyprogesterone (MPA) can be used to regularize periods and for withdrawal bleed for women who do not want to take COCP, or if COCP is contraindicated. It suppresses LH and increases testosterone clearance (liver enzyme induction). However, it can be counterproductive as it causes decrease in SHBG and therefore can increase serum free testosterone levels.

The other drugs used in the treatment of hirsutism are:

- Gonadotrophin-releasing hormone agonist (GnRH): it suppresses LH and therefore reduces ovarian androgen production. Its use is limited to short-term therapy and long-term therapy would need add back therapy with oestrogens in view of its side effects (menopausal symptoms and osteoporosis). It has no therapeutic advantage over COCP and other antiandrogens. Therefore, its use should be limited to patients with severe forms of hyperandrogenemia (e.g. ovarian hyperthecosis who do not respond to COCP or anti-androgens).

- Cyproterone acetate: it is a synthetic derivative of 17-hydroxyprogesterone. It antagonizes androgen receptor and has weak progestational and glucocorticoid activity. It suppresses actions of both testosterone and its metabolite dihydrotestosterone on tissues by blocking androgen receptors. It also suppresses LH, which in turn reduces testosterone levels. The pharmacological actions of this drug are mainly attributed to the acetate form (cyproterone acetate has three times the anti-androgenic activity of cyproterone). Side effects include mastalgia, weight gain and fluid retention causing oedema and fatigue e.g. Dianette. In high doses (200–300 mg/day) it can cause liver toxicity; hence liver enzymes should be monitored. However, low doses (2 mg) used in gynaecology are unlikely to cause any major problem.
- Flutamide: it is an anti-androgen that acts at the receptor level. It acts directly on the hair follicle and has few side effects. These include hepatotoxicity and dry skin. Like finasteride, it should be used with caution with a male fetus.
- Finasteride: it is an anti-androgen that is rarely used in the management of hirsutism. It inhibits 5-alpha reductase activity and therefore blocks the conversion of testosterone to dihydrotestosterone. However, it should be used with caution with a male fetus as it can cause demasculinization.
- Ketoconazole: is a synthetic imidazole derivative (anti-fungal agent). It decreases testosterone, androstenedione and DHEAS levels progressively over a period of time while 17 α-hydroxyprogesterone levels are increased (causes steroidogenic blockade at the level of C17-20 lyase). The side effects include liver dysfunction and therefore liver enzymes should be monitored during its use.
- Spironolactone: it is a potassium-sparing diuretic and therefore can cause hyperkalaemia and hypotension. It has a variable effect on the ovaries and adrenals: it mainly reduces androstenedione. It causes competitive inhibition of 5-alpha reductase. The side effects include fatigue and increased frequency of micturition.
- Eflornithine hydrochloride (Vaniqa cream) inhibits the enzyme (ornithine decarboxylase) in the dermal papillae required for hair growth. It slows hair growth and makes them soft when applied locally twice daily. It is recommended for facial hair but can cause acne as it blocks the glands.

Women should also be offered cosmetic approaches for hair removal. These include laser, electrolysis (permanent treatments), chemical depilatories, bleaching, waxing, tweezing, and mechanical epilators (temporary treatments).

Further reading

Collins S, Arulkumaran S, et al. *Oxford Handbook of Obstetrics & Gynaecology*. 3rd ed. Oxford: Oxford University Press; 2013.

Bader T. *OB/GYN Secrets*. 3rd ed. Maryland Heights: Mosby; 2004.

18A: False – PID is ascending infection of the upper genital tract (endometrium, tubes and ovaries and the surrounding peritoneum). The most common causative organism of PID is *Chlamydia trachomatis*. The actual prevalence of PID is difficult to ascertain as many women who have the condition may be asymptomatic (chlamydia can remain silent for years). The incidence is about 1–2% in sexually active women. If PID spreads to the upper peritoneum, it can cause perihepatic adhesions. This condition is known as Fitz-Hugh-Curtis syndrome.

18B: False – PID is more common in younger women. The risk factors for PID include:

- Women <25 years of age
- Recent sexual encounter with new partner
- History of multiple partners
- Women with prior history of PID

18C: True
18D: True
18E: True – The following factors can precipitate PID:

- Previous episode of PID
- Sex during menses
- Vaginal douching
- Bacterial vaginosis
- Uterine instrumentation (e.g. IUD)

Further reading

Collins S, Arulkumaran S, et al. *Oxford Handbook of Obstetrics & Gynaecology.* 3rd ed. Oxford: Oxford University Press; 2013.

19A: True
19B: True
19C: True
19D: False
19E: False

Most women with PID can be treated in an outpatient setting

Oral ofloxacin 400 mg twice a day plus oral metronidazole 400 mg twice a day for 14 days; or IM ceftriaxone 250 mg or IM cefoxitin 2 g immediately plus oral probenecid 1 g followed by oral doxycycline 100 mg twice a day plus oral metronidazole 400 mg twice a day for 14 days.

Antibiotic regimens are designed to cover chlamydia and gonorrhoea as well as anaerobes, gram-negative aerobes and streptococci.

The indications for hospitalization in a woman with PID include:

- Need for intravenous antibiotics
- Inability to tolerate oral medication
- If the diagnosis is uncertain
- Temperature over 38.5°C
- Evidence of tubo-ovarian abscess on ultrasound scan
- If the woman is pregnant
- Lack of response to oral therapy
- HIV/AIDS
- If the woman is not compliant

- If there are signs of peritonism
- If there is an intrauterine device in place and develops PID

The other important aspects of treatment include:

- Test for other sexually transmitted infections (STIs) including HIV, and hepatitis B and C
- Contact tracing and treatment of all partners
- Intercourse should be avoided during the course of treatment
- Drainage of pus may be required by laparoscopy if there is evidence of tubo-ovarian abscess

Further reading

Collins S, Arulkumaran S, et al. *Oxford Handbook of Obstetrics & Gynaecology*. 3rd ed. Oxford: Oxford University Press; 2013.

20A: False
20B: False
20C: True
20D: True
20E: False

Long-term consequences of PID

- Primary or secondary infertility due to tubal damage with peritubal plus ovarian adhesions
- Chronic pelvic pain
- Chronic PID
- Acute exacerbations of chronic PID
- Increased risk of ectopic pregnancy
- Potential transmission of sexually transmitted diseases to other sexual partners

Take-home messages to avoid long-term sequel or while treating women with PID

- Initiate treatment as soon as possible
- High index of suspicion is important in diagnosis to help prevent the long-term consequences of PID
- Consider PID in all young sexually active women of reproductive age who present with bilateral lower abdominal pain unless proven otherwise
- Rule out pregnancy before initiating treatment
- Reassess 48–72 hours to assure response
- Treat all sexual partners
- Encourage barrier methods of contraception even if the woman is taking COCP
- Screen and treat for other STIs when PID diagnosed

Further reading

Collins S, Arulkumaran S, et al. *Oxford Handbook of Obstetrics & Gynaecology*. 3rd ed. Oxford: Oxford University Press; 2013.

21A: False – It is required to rule out pregnancy before initiating treatment for PID but not required for diagnosing PID.

21B: True

21C: True

21D: False – A high vaginal swab (HVS) is performed for wet mount and also for culture and sensitivity of organisms.

21E: True

Investigations for diagnosing PID

- History: women usually present with lower abdominal pain often beginning, during or after menstrual period, worsening during coitus (dyspareunia); pain can be bilateral. Other associated symptoms include vaginal discharge, fever, loss of appetite, vomiting, urethritis, proctitis and intermenstrual bleeding (abnormal uterine bleeding is seen in one third of patients).
- Clinical examination
    - General examination may reveal raised temperature (50%) and tachycardia
    - Abdominal examination may reveal
        - Diffuse tenderness greatest in the lower quadrants
        - Rebound tenderness
        - Tenderness in the right upper quadrant → perihepatitis
    - Speculum exam may reveal
    - Mucopurulent discharge from the cervix
    - Pelvic examination may reveal
        - Cervical excitation
        - Adnexal tenderness
        - Adnexal mass if there is tubo-ovarian abscess

- Blood tests: WBC, CRP and blood culture if spiking >38°C
- Swabs: endocervical and high vaginal swabs
- Scans: ultrasound scan (USS) to rule tubo-ovarian abscess
- Laparoscopy: laparoscopy is the gold standard as it provides direct visualization of the pelvic organs but is not required in all cases because the diagnosis can be made clinically.
- Indications for laparoscopy include:
    - Sick patient with high suspicion of PID but an alternative condition cannot be ruled out on examination e.g. appendicitis
    - Acutely ill patient who has failed outpatient treatment for PID
    - Any patient not clearly improving after approximately 72 hours of inpatient treatment for PID
- The ultrasound scan shows a large tubo-ovarian abscess

Further reading

Collins S, Arulkumaran S, et al. *Oxford Handbook of Obstetrics & Gynaecology.* 3rd ed. Oxford: Oxford University Press; 2013.

22A: True – Symptoms include cervicitis, vaginitis and urethritis.

22B: True

22C: False
22D: True
22E: False – Can be associated with other sexually transmitted infections but in itself does not cause pelvic infection.

Infections Causing Vaginitis and Vaginal Discharge

Pathology	Physiological	Candida	Bacterial Vaginosis	Trichomonas
Appearance of vaginal discharge	Clear/creamy (cyclical)	Thick white 'cottage cheese'	Thin, grey/white	Frothy green
Odour	Nil	Nil	Fishy malodour	Fishy malodour
Associated symptoms	Nil	Itchy, sore, vulval fissures and oedema	Nil	Itchy, sore vulvovaginitis, dysuria
pH (normal 4.5)	≤4.5	≤4.5	>4.5	>4.5
Investigation		Culture from HVS or wet-mount slide showing spores and pseudohyphe	Wet mount showing clue cells and culture from HVS	Wet mount showing flagellated protozoa or culture from HVS
Treatment	Reassure	Clotrimazole 500 mg as vaginal pessary or Clotrimazole 1% cream twice daily for 7–10days	Metronidazole 400 mg orally, twice daily for 7 days or 2 g stat (avoid in first trimester of pregnancy)	Metronidazole 400 mg orally, twice daily for 7 days or 2 g stat (avoid in first trimester of pregnancy)

Further reading

Collins S, Arulkumaran S, et al. *Oxford Handbook of Obstetrics & Gynaecology.* 3rd ed. Oxford: Oxford University Press; 2013.

23A: False – Chlamydia is the most common STI in the UK.
23B: False – Herpes simplex type 1 is second most common STI and gonorrhoea is the third most common STI in the UK.
23C: True – Trichomoniasis is associated with increased risk of transmission of HIV.
23D: True
23E: True

Further reading

Collins S, Arulkumaran S, et al. *Oxford Handbook of Obstetrics & Gynaecology.* 3rd ed. Oxford: Oxford University Press; 2013.

24A: False
24B: False
24C: True
24D: True
24E: True

- Syphilis is caused by spirochaete *Treponema pallidum* and is relatively rare in the UK.
- Women with syphilis can present in three stages.
  - Primary syphilis: the incubation period is 10–90 days post-infection and can present with painless genital ulcer and inguinal lymphadenopathy.
  - Secondary syphilis: this can occur within the first 2 years of infection and can present with generalized polymorphic rash affecting palms and soles, generalized lymphadenopathy, genital condyloma lata and anterior uveitis.
  - Tertiary syphilis: 40% of people infected for over 2 years present with this condition (neurosyphilis, cardiovascular syphilis, and gummata).
- Diagnosis: rapid plasma reagin test, swab from primary lesion may demonstrate spirochaetes on dark field microscopy, fluorescent treponemal antibody absorption test (FTA-abs is most sensitive).
- Treatment: *Treponema pallidum* is sensitive to penicillin, doxycycline and erythromycin. Doxycycline is contraindicated during pregnancy.

Further reading

Collins S, Arulkumaran S, et al. *Oxford Handbook of Obstetrics & Gynaecology*. 3rd ed. Oxford: Oxford University Press; 2013.

25A: False
25B: True
25C: True
25D: False – Women with HPV infection are often asymptomatic.
25E: True

Human papillomavirus (HPV)

Subtypes 6 and 11 cause genital warts (condylomata acuminata).
Subtypes 16 and 18 are associated with CIN and cervical cancer.

- Symptoms: genital warts are often asymptomatic.
- Diagnosis: characteristic appearance of genital warts, cervical cytology to detect preinvasive conditions of cervix, HPV testing and colposcopy.
- Complications: subtypes 16 and 18 are associated with CIN and cervical cancer; smoking and immunosuppression further increases the risk.
- Treatment: physical and pharmacological destruction of warts, podophyllin application, podophyllotoxin solution, trichloroacitic acid, cryotherapy and surgery.

Further reading

Collins S, Arulkumaran S, et al. *Oxford Handbook of Obstetrics & Gynaecology*. 3rd ed. Oxford: Oxford University Press; 2013.

26A: False – About 1 in 800 women in the general population may have BRCA1 mutation and somewhat less than this may have BRCA2 mutation, which further varies with ethnic population and geographical location (e.g. about 1 in 50 Ashkenazi Jews carry these mutations). The presence of BRCA1 or BRCA2 equally increases the risk of developing breast cancer by 40–85% during lifetime depending on the population. Risk reducing measures (bilateral prophylactic mastectomy and breast reconstruction) will reduce this risk to <5%. The risk of ovarian cancer is higher with BRCA1 compared to BRCA2.

- BRCA1 and BRCA2 mutation
  - Overall these account for 3% of ovarian tumour cases (5% <40).

- Are associated with 10–50% lifetime risk of developing ovarian tumour (50% with BRCA1 and 30% with BRCA2 gene). This risk begins around the age of 40 years. Risk reducing measures (RRM) and screening methods should be discussed with these women (prophylactic oophorectomy or transvaginal scan and CA-125).

26B: True – PCOS is the only anovulatory condition associated with hyperoestrogenemia. It therefore increases the overall risk of endometrial hyperplasia and endometrial cancer. Women with PCOS are generally obese, which further adds to the risk (the adipose tissue in the body converts androgens to oestrogens by aromatization and therefore contributes further to the hyperoestrogenic milieu). In view of this, the first line of management in women with PCOS is lifestyle changes (weight loss).

- The other conditions where unopposed oestrogen stimulation of the endometrium occurs include:
  - Obesity
  - Oestrogen-producing ovarian tumours like granulosa cell tumours
  - Oestrogen-only hormone replacement therapy (HRT) or combined HRT for long term

- Liver cirrhosis (oestrogen is metabolized in the liver. If there is any disruption of the pathway, the metabolism is affected and increases the serum oestrogen levels)

26C: False – Induction of ovulation with clomiphene does not increase the risk of endometrial cancer. However, when it is used for more than 12 cycles it has possibly shown to increase the risk of ovarian cancer (limited evidence).

26D: False – Tamoxifen has been used for ovulation induction in women who are sensitive to clomiphene citrate. When used for ovulation induction, there is no risk of endometrial cancer. Tamoxifen is an oestrogen antagonist on breast and oestrogen agonist on the endometrium. It is used for pre-menopausal women in the treatment of breast cancer when the tumour is oestrogen-receptor positive. This is generally advised for 5 years and has been shown to reduce the risk of recurrence of breast cancer by 50%. However, because of its agonist action on the endometrium, it can cause endometrial hyperplasia and subsequently endometrial cancer. This effect can occur any time but mainly when it is used for longer than 5 years.

26E: True – HNPCC is a genetic disorder that runs in families and affects the ability of people to repair their own DNA. It therefore increases the risk of colon cancer and also increases the risk of endometrial, ovarian and stomach cancer.

Further reading

Cook LS, Nelson HE, et al. Endometrial cancer and a family history of cancer. *Gynecol Oncol*. 2013; 130(2):334–339.

Collins S, Arulkumaran S, et al. *Oxford Handbook of Obstetrics & Gynaecology*. 3rd ed. Oxford: Oxford University Press; 2013.

27A: True
27B: True
27C: False
27D: False – Women in the menopause have amenorrhoea. They can present with postmenopausal bleeding.
27E: True

Short-term symptoms/consequences

- Vasomotor symptoms (80%): hot flushes (usually due to pulsatile FSH release in increased amounts leading to peripheral vasodilatation), night sweats (4–5 years)
- Sleep disturbance
- Sexual dysfunction: vaginal dryness, due to decreased levels of oestrogen, decreased levels of androgen. Therefore, low sexual desire and painful sex (dyspareunia). This can respond well to local vaginal oestrogen cream or pessaries.
- Psychological symptoms: depression, anxiety, irritability and mood swings, lethargy and lack of energy.

Further reading

Collins S, Arulkumaran S, et al. *Oxford Handbook of Obstetrics & Gynaecology*. 3rd ed. Oxford: Oxford University Press; 2013.

28A: False – Primary osteoporosis due to ageing and decreased oestrogen levels.
28B: True
28C: False – Urogenital atrophy.
28D: True
28E: True

Menopause is defined as the absence of periods for more than a year.

Pathophysiology of normal menstrual cycle and menopause: gradual depletion of functioning ovarian follicles, decrease in inhibin levels from granulosa cells, increase in FSH production from pituitary gland, accelerated follicular phase, increase in basal estradiol levels during menstrual period, follicular cysts, granulosa cells loose ability to produce estradiol, FSH increases (LH increases).

After menopause there is a greater decline in estradiol levels, higher androgen-to-oestrogen ratio, and oestrogen is mainly produced in adipose tissue by aromatization of androstenedione and testosterone.

Long-Term Consequences of Menopause

Sign	Symptom	Cause	Other Risk Factors	Treatment
Primary osteoporosis (1 in 3 women) due to decreased BMD	Fractures (common sites include lower end of radius, proximal femur and vertebrae)	Oestrogen deficiency and ageing	Genetic Constitutional ((↓BMI, early menopause) Lifestyle (smoking, alchohol abuse) Dietary (decreased calcium intake) Medical conditions (hyperthyroidism, malabsorption syndrome, chronic liver disease) Premature menopause or premature ovarian failure	Calcium Biphosphonates HRT during the window period (50–60 years of age)
↑ risk of cardiovascular disease (CVD) and stroke	IHD Myocardial infarction Stroke	Partly due to oestrogen deficiency	Genetic, ↑ BMI, smoking, hypercholes-terolaemia, hypertension and diabetes	Reduction of risk factors (CVD most common cause of death in women after 60)
Urogenital atrophy	**Urinary:** frequency, urgency, nocturia, incontinence, recurrent UTI **Vaginal atrophy:** dyspareunia, itching, burning and dryness	Oestrogen deficiency		Local vaginal oestrogen cream or pessaries

Further reading

Collins S, Arulkumaran S, et al. *Oxford Handbook of Obstetrics & Gynaecology.* 3rd ed. Oxford: Oxford University Press; 2013.

29A: True
29B: False
29C: True
29D: False – DEXA scan is contraindicated during pregnancy.
29E: True

Bone loss begins during menopausal transition. The decrease in bone mineral density (BMD) can be detected by a DEXA scan. This is a special X-ray to determine a person's bone mineral density. It compares a person's bone density with the bone density of a young healthy adult or an adult of one's own age, gender and ethnicity. The difference is then calculated as a standard deviation (SD). The difference between a person's measurement and that of a young adult is known as the T score, and the difference between the same person's measurement and that of someone of the same age is known as the Z score.

Uses of DEXA scan

- Most commonly used to diagnose osteoporosis (compromised bone mineral density)
- Can be used to detect osteopenia (very low mineral density)
- Can also help to detect osteomalacia (softening of bones caused by vitamin D deficiency)

WHO Osteoporosis Classification

Diagnosis	T scores
Normal	Above −1.0 SD
Osteopenia	Between < −1.0 and > −2.5 SD
Osteoporosis	Below −2.5 SD
Severe osteoporosis	Below −2.5 SD plus fragility fractures
A Z score below −2 SD indicates that bone mineral density is lower than expected for that age (in premenopausal women this should trigger a search for an underlying cause).	

- Cannot predict of likelihood of fracture

Further reading

Collins S, Arulkumaran S, et al. *Oxford Handbook of Obstetrics & Gynaecology.* 3rd ed. Oxford: Oxford University Press; 2013.

30A: False
30B: True
30C: False
30D: True
30E: True

Premature menopause is defined as menopause before the age of 40 (occurs in 1% of women below the age of 40 and 0.1% below the age of 30 years).

- Aetiology
  - Unknown in most cases
  - Primary causes: chromosome abnormalities, FSH receptor gene polymorphism, inhibin B mutation, enzyme deficiencies (galactosaemia), autoimmune disease
  - Secondary causes: chemotherapy, radiotherapy, bilateral oopherectomy or surgical menopause, history of hysterectomy, infection (e.g. mumps)

- Clinical presentation
  - Secondary amenorrhoea or oligomenorrhoea is the most common presentation
- Co-existing conditions
  - Hypothyroidism
  - Addison's disease
  - Diabetes mellitus
  - Chromosome abnormalities
- Consequences
  - Increased risk of osteoporosis
  - Cardiovascular disease
  - Psychological trauma
  - Lower risk of breast malignancy
- Management issues
  - Reduced fertility, may require assisted conception, need for contraception if no fertility goals as there is risk of sporadic ovulation
  - Oestrogen replacement (HRT) needed until average age of natural menopause
- Psychological counselling

Further reading

Collins S, Arulkumaran S, et al. *Oxford Handbook of Obstetrics & Gynaecology.* 3rd ed. Oxford: Oxford University Press; 2013.

31A: False – Fluid in endometrial cavity in postmenopausal women is associated with malignancy.
31B: False – Hysteroscopy fails to detect endometrial pathology in less then 1% of cases.
31C: False – Only 10% of the women with postmenopausal bleeding will have endometrial cancer while 80–88% of women will have atrophic endometrium. In view of the 10% risk of endometrial cancer, all women with PMB should be referred urgently to rapid access gynaeoncology clinic and should be seen in the clinic within 2 weeks of referral.
31D: True
31E: False

Further reading

NICE clinical guideline 27. *Referral guidelines for suspected cancer.* 2005. Available at: publications.nice.org.uk/referral-guidelines-for-suspected-cancer-cg27

Rogerson L, Jones S. The investigation of women with postmenopausal bleeding. Pacc reviews no 98/07. RCOG Press; 2003. pp 10–13.

Sahdev A. Imaging the endometrium in postmenopausal bleeding. *BMJ.* 2007; 24; 334(7594): 635–636.

32A: False
32B: False
32C: False

32D: False
32E: True

Further reading

Collins S, Arulkumaran S, et al. *Oxford Handbook of Obstetrics & Gynaecology.* 3rd ed. Oxford: Oxford University Press; 2013.

33A: False – Transvaginal scan is good enough to differentiate between benign and malignant cysts.
33B: True – If the ovarian cyst is unilateral and unilocular with low RMI (<25), postmenopausal women with ovarian cyst can either be managed conservatively or removed surgically. Both options can be discussed with the patient and it should be an informed choice.
33C: True – If the postmenopausal woman opts for conservative management of the ovarian cyst, she will need a repeat transvaginal scan and CA-125 every 3–4 months. If the cyst remains the same or decreases in size, she can be discharged to her GP at the end of one year. If the cyst increases in size during follow up, it warrants surgical removal
33D: False – Ultrasound guided aspiration of the cyst in postmenopausal women is not recommended by the RCOG.
33E: True – With the above findings, the likelihood of the cyst being benign is high; therefore, laparoscopic oophorectomy is an acceptable treatment.
RMI is calculated by multiplying these three parameters:

1. Ultrasound (USG) features (U = 0 for USG score of 0, U = 1 for USG score of 1 and U = 3 for USG score of 2–5)
2. Menopausal status (use 3 for postmenopausal women and 1 for premenopausal women)
3. CA-125 levels (actual value from the blood test)

The final number acquired after multiplication of the above factors is regarded as the RMI. This number determines the risk of ovarian cancer e.g. RMI <25 is considered low risk and the risk of cancer is <3%, RMI 25–250 is considered moderate risk and the risk of cancer is 20%, and RMI >250 is considered high risk for malignancy and the risk of cancer is 75%.

Further reading

RCOG Green-top guideline No. 34. *Ovarian cysts in postmenopausal women.* 2003. Available at: www.rcog.org.uk/womens-health/clinical-guidance /ovarian-cysts-postmenopausal-women-green-top-34

NICE clinical guideline No. 122. *Ovarian cancer: the recognition and initial management.* 2011. Available at: publications.nice.org.uk/ovarian-cancer-cg122

Collins S, Arulkumaran S, et al. *Oxford Handbook of Obstetrics & Gynaecology.* 3rd ed. Oxford: Oxford University Press; 2013.

34A: False – Simple hyperplasia without atypia has low risk of malignancy (1%) and therefore can be managed conservatively with progestogens. Simple hyperplasia with atypia has 8% risk of endometrial malignancy and can be treated with high-dose progestogens. This should be followed by hysteroscopy and endometrial biopsy in 3 months.

34B: True – Complex hyperplasia without atypia confers a 3% risk of malignancy while complex hyperplasia with atypia has 30–50% risk of malignancy.

34C: True – There is a very high risk of coexistent endometrial cancer (25–50%) associated with complex endometrial atypical hyperplasia and therefore total abdominal hysterectomy and bilateral salpingo-oophorectomy is recommended in such women.

34D: False

34E: True – The treatment options are determined by the histology. The treatment options include:

- Weight loss if high BMI
- Progestogens: oral/Mirena IUS
- Repeat hysteroscopy and endometrial biopsy in 3 months
- Offer hysterectomy and bilateral salpingo-ooprectomy

Further reading

Collins S, Arulkumaran S, et al. *Oxford Handbook of Obstetrics & Gynaecology.* 3rd ed. Oxford: Oxford University Press; 2013.

13

FERTILITY CONTROL (CONTRACEPTION AND TERMINATION OF PREGNANCY) – QUESTIONS

SBAs

Question 1

Which one of the following is true with regard to the use of emergency contraception (EC)?

A. Ulipristal acetate/ellaOne is licensed for EC up to 3 days of unprotected sexual intercourse (UPSI).
B. Oral levonorgestrel/levonelle is effective for up to 5 days of UPSI.
C. Mirena IUS inserted within 5 days of UPSI is a highly efficacious form of EC.
D. Levonelle cannot be used more than once in a cycle.
E. Levonelle and ellaone are equally efficacious.

Question 2

With regard to contraception and breastfeeding, which one of the following statements is true?

A. The hormonal method of contraception is not recommended during breastfeeding.
B. IUD can be inserted anytime within the first 6 weeks after delivery in breastfeeding women.
C. Lactational amenorrhoea method is >98% effective in women who are fully breastfeeding within the first 6 months.
D. COCP need not be avoided during breastfeeding.
E. Progesterone-only implants are not recommended in the first 6 months postpartum.

Question 3

With regard to missed contraceptive pills, which one of the following statements is false?

A. Additional contraception is not required if one active COCP pill is missed.
B. Additional protection for 7 days is recommended if two active COCP pills are missed.
C. Missed pill is defined as one that is more than 12 hours late from the time it should have been taken.
D. Additional contraception is needed for 48 hours if one POP pill is missed.
E. Additional contraception is need if the COCP is started after day 5 of the menstrual cycle.

Question 4

With regard to POPs, which one of the following statements is true?

A. Contraindicated in women with undiagnosed vaginal bleeding
B. Contraindicated in women with recent history of breast cancer
C. Act mainly by suppressing ovulation
D. Contraindicated in smokers over the age of 40 years
E. Efficacy decreases with age

Question 5

With regard to Mirena IUS, which one of the following is true?

A. Contraindicated in nulliparous women
B. Contains 52 micrograms of etonogestrel
C. Associated with an increased risk of pelvic infection
D. Can be used with oestrogen replacement therapy for endometrial protection
E. Cannot be used to treat endometriosis

Question 6

With regard to progestogen-only implants, which one of the following is true?

A. Act primarily by altering the cervical mucus
B. Licensed for 5 years of continuous use
C. Return of fertility is delayed for 6 months
D. Altered bleeding pattern is a common side effect
E. Contraindicated in women with BMI >30

Question 7

A 25-year-old woman who was recently diagnosed with trophoblastic disease is being followed up at the referral centre. Which one of the following is incorrect advice to give?

A. Advise against conception until follow up is complete.
B. IUD is contraindicated until hCG levels normalize.
C. Outcome of all subsequent pregnancies should be notified to the screening centre.
D. COCP may be used after hCG levels normalize.
E. Barrier contraceptive methods can only be used after hCG levels normalize.

Question 8

With respect to recurrent miscarriages, which one of the following is true?

A. Women with recurrent miscarriages should be screened routinely for thyroid antibodies.
B. Antiphospholipid syndrome is the most important treatable cause of recurrent miscarriages.
C. Recurrent miscarriage is when there is a loss of two or more consecutive pregnancies.
D. Pelvic ultrasound is not indicated in all cases.
E. Low-dose aspirin plus heparin are of no proven benefit in improving the pregnancy outcome in women with antiphospholipid syndrome.

Question 9

You are reviewing the investigation results of a couple with primary subfertility. Which one of the following components of semen analysis is abnormal?

A. Volume: 4 ml
B. Liquefaction time: 20 minutes
C. Concentration: 40 million/ml
D. Motility: 20% motile
E. Morphology: 50% normal forms

Question 10

Which one of the following statements is not true with respect to BMI and fertility?

A. Women with BMI ≥30 are likely to take longer to conceive.
B. BMI ≥30 in men has no effect on fertility outcomes.
C. Women with BMI <19 and irregular menstruation are likely to improve their chance of conception by weight gain.
D. Women with BMI ≥30 and who are not ovulating are likely to improve their chances of conception by losing weight.
E. Women with BMI ≥30 prior to assisted reproductive techniques are likely to have less success rates.

Question 11

Which one of the following statements is true regarding emergency contraception with levonorgestrel (1.5 mg)?

A. Single dose provides cover for the rest of the menstrual cycle
B. Can be used only once during any menstrual cycle
C. Efficacy remains the same when used up to 120 hours after unprotected sexual intercourse
D. Recommended dose is to take two tablets of levonorgestrel (1.5 mg) to achieve better efficacy
E. If a woman vomits within 2 hours of ingestion of levonorgestrel (1.5 mg), then the recommendation is to take another pill of levonorgestrel (1.5 mg)

EMQs

OPTIONS FOR QUESTIONS 1–3

A. Additional contraception for 7 days
B. Additional contraception for 14 days
C. No need for additional contraception
D. Emergency contraception
E. Take missed pill as soon as possible
F. Have the usual 7-day break
G. No need for emergency contraception
H. Additional contraception for next 48 hours
I. Leave the missed pills
J. Omit pill free interval

Instructions

For each clinical scenario below, choose the single most appropriate contraceptive advice from the above list of options. Each option may be used once, more than once or not at all.

1. A 22-year-old woman attends the family planning clinic for advice after she missed her Cerazette pill. After realizing the mishap, she takes the missed pill approximately 42 hours after the last pill. You have advised her to take the next pill at the usual time and one of the above options.
2. A 30-year-old woman attends the family planning clinic for removal of Nexaplanon due to irregular bleeding patterns and she wishes to start combined oral contraceptive pills. You have advised her to start taking the pills from that day onwards and one of the above options.
3. A 32-year-old woman attends the family planning clinic for advice on additional contraception after an episode of detachment of combined transdermal patch for >48 hours. She had worn the patch continuously for 7 days prior the detachment and there was no history of unprotected sexual intercourse during the patch-free period. You have informed her that there is no need for emergency contraception and one of the options above.

OPTIONS FOR QUESTIONS 4–6

A. Combined oral contraceptive pills (COCP)
B. Vaginal ring
C. Intrauterine device (IUD)
D. Barrier methods
E. Progestogen-only pills (POP)
F. Hysteroscopic sterilization
G. Oestrogen patch
H. Depo-Provera
I. Mirena intrauterine system
J. Progestogen implant

Instructions

For each clinical scenario below, choose the single most appropriate contraceptive method from the above list of options. Each option may be used once, more than once or not at all.

4. A 33-year-old para 3, HIV positive woman on antiretroviral therapy seeks your advice on the most effective emergency contraceptive method after an episode of condom mishap. She is otherwise clinically well.

5. A 34-year-old woman comes to see you urgently after coming from a holiday with a history of unprotected sexual intercourse (UPSI) and missed pills on a few occasions over the last week. She has taken Ulipristal acetate after the first UPSI 6 days ago and the last UPSI was 3 days ago. Her menstrual cycles are regular at 5/28 days. She is on day 14 of her cycle and feels that this is not the right time for her to conceive, as she recently got promoted at work.

6. A 40-year-old para 2 woman with twins was readmitted with high temperature 2 weeks after an emergency caesarean section for failure to progress. She is on broad spectrum antibiotics for endometritis with good clinical improvement. She has hypertension, type 2 diabetes and had a pulmonary embolism at 32 weeks' gestation, for which she is on anticoagulants. She is struggling to cope with the twins and the multiple appointments due to her medical conditions. She wishes to have a long-term reversible contraceptive method prior to discharge.

OPTIONS FOR QUESTIONS 7–9

A. POP
B. Ulipristal
C. Levonorgestrel intrauterine system
D. Nexaplanon
E. COCP
F. Barrier contraception
G. Depo-Provera
H. Copper IUD
 I. Progestogen-only emergency contraception
J. NuvaRing

Instructions

For each clinical scenario below, choose the single most appropriate contraceptive method from the above list of options. Each option may be used once, more than once or not at all.

7. A 15-year-old girl comes to see you for reliable contraceptive advice after a condom mishap. Her menstrual cycles are irregular, heavy and painful to the extent that she had to miss school during the heavy days during the last three cycles.
8. A 38-year-old nulliparous woman seeks your advice on the most effective method of contraception after recent diagnosis of breast cancer.
9. A 20-year-old nulliparous woman attends the family planning clinic to discuss the contraceptive options that are suitable for her. She is not keen on pills or injections and had issues with compliance in the past, and doesn't like the idea of having devices in the vagina or uterus.

OPTIONS FOR QUESTIONS 10–12

A. Contraceptive vaginal ring (NuvaRing)
B. COCP
C. Copper IUD
D. Emergency contraception
E. Depomedroxyprogesterone acetate (DMPA)
F. Mirena intrauterine system (Mirena IUS)
G. Male pill
H. Microinsert sterilization device (Essure)
I. POP
J. Bilateral clipping of the fallopian tube (Sterilization)
K. Transdermal contraceptive patch (EVRA)
L. Third generation progestins
M. Bilateral ligation of vas deferens (Vasectomy)

Instructions

For each contraceptive action and uses described below, choose the most likely group of contraceptive method from the list above. Each answer can be used once, more than once or not at all.

10. This is a permanent hysteroscopic tubal sterilization device that is 99.9% effective.
11. This is an alternative form of birth control in women who cannot take oestrogen and, if the usual time of ingestion is delayed for more than 3 hours, an alternative form of birth control should be used for the following 48 hours.
12. This provides contraception for 8–10 years and, if placed within 120 hours of unprotected intercourse, can also be used as a form of emergency contraception.

OPTIONS FOR QUESTIONS 13–15

A. Acts by preventing the embryo travelling to the uterine cavity
B. Causes changes in the cervical mucus but does not cause inhibition of ovulation
C. Does not inhibit ovulation
D. Inhibits ovulation in 15% of menstrual cycles
E. Impairs sperm migration and suppresses endometrium
F. Inhibits ovulation in 99–100% of menstrual cycles
G. Inhibits ovulation in 97% of menstrual cycles
H. Inhibits ovulation in 80% of the menstrual cycles
I. Inhibits ovulation in 50–60% of menstrual cycles and also relies on other mechanisms such as alteration in the cervical mucus and endometrium
J. Inhibits ovulation in 30% of menstrual cycles and also relies on other mechanisms such as alteration in the cervical mucus and endometrium
K. Inhibits ovulation in 100% of menstrual cycles
L. Mainly prevents fertilization and also blocks implantation

Instruction

For each drug mentioned below, choose the single most appropriate mechanism of action from the above list of options. Each option may be used once, more than once or not at all.

13. Copper IUD
14. POP
15. Desogestrel

MCQs

1. With regard to contraceptive choices for young people:
    A. Young women should not be offered Mirena intrauterine system (IUS) if they are nulliparous.
    B. Age of 18 years is a contraindication for use of injectable progesterone in women (e.g. depomedroxyprogesterone acetate [DMPA]).
    C. Teenage women with learning disabilities should not be considered Fraser competent.
    D. Progestorone implants (e.g. Etonorgestrol implant) are contraindicated in young women with history of irregular periods.
    E. Intrauterine copper device (IUCD) is contraindicated in young women who are nulliparous due to risk of vasovagal shock at insertion.

2. The contraindications for combined oral contraceptive pill (COCP) use include:
    A. Migraine without aura
    B. Pregnancy
    C. Previous history of superficial thrombophlebitis
    D. Mild hypertension
    E. Overweight

3. With regard to COCP use:
    A. It regularizes the periods.
    B. It increases menstrual blood loss when used for a long period.
    C. It increases the risk of ovarian cancer.
    D. It increases the risk of endometrial cancer.
    E. It may increase the risk of breast cancer.

4. The progesterone-only pill:
    A. Can be used in women suffering from breast cancer
    B. Can be used in women with migraine
    C. Is recommended in women with current DVT
    D. Can be used in women during early postpartum period
    E. Can be used in women with hypertension

5. The failure rates of hormonal contraceptives include:
    A. COCP: 5% per 100 woman years
    B. POP: 10% per 100 woman years
    C. Progesterone injectables: 3% per 100 woman years
    D. Progesterone implants: <1% per 100 woman years
    E. Mirena IUS: 3% per 100 woman years

6. Emergency contraception (EC):
   A. Levonorgestrel 1.5 mg (oral) is the drug of choice for EC in the UK.
   B. Levonorgestrel 1.5 mg (oral) should be ideally taken after 48–72 hours following unprotected intercourse to be more effective in preventing pregnancy.
   C. Levonorgestrel 1.5 mg (oral) is not as effective when used multiple times in the same cycle following unprotected intercourse.
   D. Levonorgestrel 1.5 mg (oral) is not sold without prescription for women under 16 years of age in the UK.
   E. Copper IUD (EC) is less effective in preventing unwanted pregnancy compared to Levonorgestrel 1.5 mg (oral).

7. As per UK Medical Eligibility Criteria (UKMEC) the following are correctly matched with regard to use of COCP:
   A. Current venous thromboembolism (VTE): UK category 3
   B. History of VTE: UK category 4
   C. Migraine with aura at the age of 20: UK category 3
   D. Migraine without aura at the age of 20: UK category 4
   E. Minor surgery without immobilization: UK category 1

8. During breastfeeding:
   A. Use of oestrogen-only contraception while breastfeeding does not affect breast milk volume.
   B. Use of combination oestrogen and progestogen contraception while breastfeeding will affect the breast milk volume.
   C. Use of progestogen-only contraception while breastfeeding has been shown to affect infant growth.
   D. Exclusive breastfeeding resulting in amenorrhoea is over 98% effective in preventing pregnancy.
   E. Decrease in frequency of breastfeeding increases the risk of pregnancy.

9. With regard to advice given to women starting specific methods of contraception during the postpartum period:
   A. Contraception should be started within one week following childbirth.
   B. Contraception is not required for at least 21 days following childbirth.
   C. If a hormonal method of contraception is initiated before 21 days after childbirth, an additional contraception is required for these women.
   D. Combined hormonal contraception can be commenced before 21 days after childbirth for all women.
   E. Women who are breastfeeding should be advised to start combined hormonal contraceptive method before 21 days after childbirth.

10. During the postpartum period:
    A. Both breastfeeding and non-breastfeeding women are allowed to start POP at any time after childbirth.
    B. Breastfeeding women can start progestogen-only injectable method at any time following childbirth.
    C. Use of DMPA during early puerperium may result in heavy prolonged bleeding.
    D. Copper IUD use is contraindicated during first 21 days following childbirth.
    E. A levonorgestrel-releasing intrauterine system (LNG-IUS) can be inserted from day 28 following childbirth.

11. With regard to preconceptual advice for women with inflammatory bowel disease (IBD) planning pregnancy:
    A. If the woman is taking methotrexate for IBD, the use of contraception should be advised during and for at least 3 months after treatment.
    B. Contraception is not required for women who are taking infliximab or adalimumab.
    C. Caesarean section is the most appropriate mode of delivery following ileal pouch-anal anastomosis surgery
    D. Vaginal delivery is an absolute contraindication following ileal pouch-anal anastomosis surgery.
    E. Women with IBD should be advised to conceive when the disease is well controlled.

12. Regarding contraceptive use in women with IBD:
    A. The efficacy of contraception is decreased in women with Crohn's disease who have small bowel disease and malabsorption.
    B. The use of any contraception would exacerbate IBD.
    C. Women using COCP should use additional contraception if they are taking antibiotic courses of less than 3 weeks and for 7 days after the antibiotic has been discontinued.
    D. Women with IBD and using the COCP can continue the pill when undergoing major elective gynaecological surgery.
    E. Laparoscopic sterilization is an inappropriate method of contraception for women with IBD who have had previous pelvic or abdominal surgery.

13. With regard to the use of contraception in women with epilepsy using antiepileptic medication:
   A. It is advisable to use contraception until seizures are adequately controlled.
   B. If the woman is using hepatic enzyme-inducing drugs, low-dose combined COCPs should be used to increase the efficacy of the contraceptive pills.
   C. If the woman is using hepatic enzyme-inducing drugs, she should be warned about requiring much lower doses of progestogens to attain adequate contraception.
   D. The dose of the COCP does not need to be changed if the woman is taking enzyme-inducing antiepileptic medication.
   E. The woman would need double the normal dose of levonorgestrel for emergency contraction compared to women without epilepsy.

14. A 28-year-old para 2 woman comes to her GP for contraceptive advice. She is adamant that she wants to be sterilized. The GP should give the following advice regarding this method of contraception before referring her to a gynaecologist for surgery:
   A. It is a temporary method of contraception.
   B. The NHS does offer reversal of the sterilization operation.
   C. It can be performed by keyhole operation (laparoscopy).
   D. Alternative methods of contraception should be discussed with the patient including vasectomy for her partner.
   E. Sterilization is not 100% effective.

15. With regard to contraception for young people:
   A. COCP cannot be prescribed to a girl less than 16 years of age if Fraser competent.
   B. Depo-Provera (medroxyprogesterone acetate) injection can be administered to girls above 15 years of age on request.
   C. Depo-Provera (medroxyprogesterone acetate) injection can be administered to girls above 15 years in the presence of learning disability.
   D. If the girl is Fraser competent and requests that her parents should not be informed, confidentiality should be maintained.
   E. If she is Fraser competent and requests contraception, she doesn't need to inform her parents.

16. Regarding contraception advice the following statements are either true or false:
    A. A 29-year-old woman comes to the GP for advice regarding contraception. She had a spontaneous vaginal delivery one week ago and is very keen to breastfeed. The best option for her at this stage is the use of COCP.
    B. A 34-year-old woman comes to the GP for advice regarding her unprotected intercourse 24 hour ago. She had a spontaneous vaginal delivery 4 weeks ago and is bottle feeding her baby. Her GP suggests emergency contraception is not indicated.
    C. A 28-year-old woman comes to the GP for advice regarding long-term contraception. She had spontaneous vaginal delivery 6 weeks ago. She had unprotected intercourse 3 days ago. The best option in her case is levonorgestrel 1.5 mg single oral dose.
    D. A 39-year-old woman comes to her GP for advice regarding contraception. She had spontaneous vaginal delivery 6 weeks ago and is not keen on breastfeeding her child. She also gives a history of bloating and acne during her periods. The best option in her case is POP.
    E. A 27-year-old woman comes to her GP for advice regarding contraception. She had spontaneous vaginal delivery 8 weeks ago and was not keen on breastfeeding. She gives a history of heavy menstrual bleeding in the past. The best option for her contraceptive needs is copper IUD.

17. Depo-Provera (medroxyprogesterone acetate) injection:
    A. Is the first line of treatment for menorrhagia
    B. Is administered every 4 weeks for contraception
    C. Increases the risk of ovarian cancer
    D. Can be used as a contraceptive method in women who are breastfeeding
    E. Return of fertility is immediate following withdrawal of this method of contraception

18. With regard to the first prescription for the COCP:
    A. It can be used in women with a history of migraine with aura.
    B. It can be used in women above the age of 35 years who smoke >15 cigarettes per day.
    C. It can be used in women above the age of 40 years in the absence of other risk factors.
    D. If the pill is started on day one of the menstrual period additional contraception is required.
    E. If the pill is started on day 6 of the menstrual period additional contraception is not required.

19. With regard to emergency contraception:
    A. Levonorgestrel 0.5 mg is as effective as 1.5 mg.
    B. Levonorgestrel 1.5 mg can be taken until 5 days after unprotected sexual intercourse.
    C. Levonorgestrel 1.5 mg is more effective than copper IUD when used for emergency contraception.
    D. Copper IUD is more effective than Mirena IUS for emergency contraception.
    E. Copper IUD used for emergency contraception can be continued if the woman wants to use it for long-term contraception.

20. With regard to termination of pregnancy (abortion):
    A. At 10 weeks' gestation, it can be performed under general anaesthesia if the woman requesting is on a regular 28-day cycle.
    B. Terminations up to 9 weeks' gestation can be performed using medical methods.
    C. It can be offered up to a maximum of 13 weeks' gestation in the best interest of the patient's mental and physical wellbeing if continuation of pregnancy is likely to deteriorate her condition.
    D. The signature of two medical practitioners is necessary for the legal authorization of abortion.
    E. Abortion is illegal in Northern Ireland.

14

FERTILITY CONTROL (CONTRACEPTION AND TERMINATION OF PREGNANCY) – ANSWERS

SBAs

Answer 1: E

Oral levonorgestrel (LNG), oral ulipristal acetate and copper IUD are forms of EC, but not Mirena IUS. LNG EC is taken as a single dose of 1500 micrograms (mcg) as soon as possible or within 72 hours of unprotected coitus, which is highly efficacious and prevents ~85% of expected pregnancies. It can be used more than once in a cycle if clinically indicated. Single dose of Ulipristal acetate 30 mg is licensed for EC up to 120 hours after UPSI; it is as efficacious as LNG EC but not recommended more than once in a cycle. Copper IUD works by inhibiting fertilization by causing direct toxicity and is 99% effective, if given within 5 days of unprotected coitus.

Further reading

FSRH clinical effectiveness unit guidance. *Emergency contraception.* Available at: www.fsrh.org/pages/Clinical_Guidance_2.asp

Answer 2: C

Lactational amenorrhoea method is >98% effective in preventing pregnancy in women who are <6 months postpartum, fully breastfeeding and amenorrhoeic. Hormonal contraception is not contraindicated during breastfeeding. Progestogen-only preparations (pills, injectables, implants) can be commenced at any time, whereas COCP is contraindicated in breastfeeding women within the first 6 weeks after delivery but not 6 months after delivery. Intrauterine devices and systems can be inserted anytime at or after 4 weeks or within the first 48 hours of delivery, whether breastfeeding or not. It is not advised between 48 hours and 4 weeks postpartum because of the increased risk of uterine perforation.

Further reading

FSRH medical eligibility criteria. *Summary sheets: common reversible methods*. 2009. Available at: www.fsrh.org/pdfs/ukmecsummarysheets2009.pdf

Answer 3: C

Missed pill is defined as one that is more than 24 hours late from the time it should have been taken. Additional contraception is needed if the COCP is started later than day 5 of the menstrual cycle or when two or more pills are missed, but not when one pill is missed. If one POP is missed, then additional contraception is needed for 48 hours.

Further reading

FSRH clinical effectiveness unit guidance. *Missed pill recommendations*. 2011. Available at: www.fsrh.org/pdfs/CEUStatementMissedPills.pdf

Answer 4: B

POPs act mainly by inducing cervical mucus hostility and interfering with ovarian hormonal function without necessarily suppressing ovulation. Efficacy increases with age and POPs are suitable for women with hypertension, diabetes, BMI >35 and in women who smoke >15 cigarettes per day and contraindicated only in women with current or recent history of breast cancer.

Further reading

FSRH clinical effectiveness unit guidance. *Progestogen-only pills*. 2009. Available at: www.fsrh.org/pdfs/CEUGuidanceProgestogenOnlyPill09.pdf

Answer 5: D

Mirena IUS contains 52 mg of levonorgestrel and is a long-acting reversible contraceptive method, licensed for 5 years of contraception. It is the recommended first-line treatment for heavy menstrual bleeding and can be used to treat endometriosis and dysmenorrhoea. It can also be used, along with oestrogen replacement therapy, for endometrial protection. It is protective against pelvic infection due to its progestogenic effect on cervical mucus.

Further reading

FSRH clinical effectiveness unit guidance. *Intrauterine contraception*. 2007. Available at: www.fsrh.org/pdfs/CEUGuidanceIntrauterineContraceptionNov07.pdf

Answer 6: D

Progesterone-only implant is a very effective method of contraception with a <1 in 1000 over 3 years failure rate. They primarily act by preventing ovulation. Women with a BMI of more than 30 can use progesterone-only implants without any restriction. Irregular bleeding pattern is the most common side effect, occurring in almost 50% of women, and there is no evidence of a delay in return of fertility following removal.

Further reading

FSRH clinical effectiveness unit guidance. *Progestogen-only implants*. 2008. Available at: www.fsrh.org/pdfs/CEUGuidanceProgestogenOnlyImplantsApril08.pdf

Answer 7: E

Women with trophoblastic disease should be advised to use barrier methods of contraception until hCG levels revert to normal.

Further reading

RCOG Green-top guideline No. 38. *Gestational trophoblastic disease*. 2010. Available at: www.rcog.org.uk/womens-health/clinical-guidance /management-gestational-trophoblastic-neoplasia-green-top-38

Answer 8: B

Recurrent miscarriage is when there is loss of three or more consecutive pregnancies. All women with recurrent miscarriages should be screened for antiphospholipid antibodies as antiphospholipid syndrome is the most common treatable cause of recurrent miscarriages. Pelvic ultrasound, thrombophilia screen, cytogenetic analysis of products of conception of the third and subsequent miscarriages should be performed routinely, but not thyroid antibodies. Low-dose aspirin and heparin improve the pregnancy outcome in women with antiphospholipid antibodies.

Further reading

RCOG Green-top guideline No. 17. *Recurrent miscarriage, investigation and treatment of couples*. 2011. Available at: www.rcog.org.uk/womens-health/clinical-guidance /investigation-and-treatment-couples-recurrent-miscarriage-green-top-17

Answer 9: D

WHO standards for 'normal' semen analysis include semen volume of 2–5 ml, liquefaction time <30min, concentration of 20–200 million/ml, greater than 40% normal morphology and >40% motility with white cells <1 million/ml.

Further reading

Collins S, Arulkumaran S, et al. *Oxford Handbook of Obstetrics & Gynaecology*. 3rd ed. Oxford: Oxford University Press; 2013.

Answer 10: B

Men with BMI ≥30 are likely to have reduced fertility.

Further reading

NICE clinical guideline 156. *Fertility*. 2013. Available at: www.nice.org.uk /nicemedia/live/14078/62769/62769.pdf

Answer 11: E

Levonorgestrel (1.5 mg): oral

- Single dose is the recommended dose unless the woman is taking liver enzyme induction medications.
- If taken within 72 hours of unprotected sexual intercourse, 85% of pregnancies are prevented.
- It may be used up to 120 hours after unprotected sexual intercourse (UPSI), but the efficacy is uncertain.
- It may be used more than once in one menstrual cycle.
- It does not provide contraceptive cover for the rest of the menstrual cycle.
- Side effects: nausea, vomiting and erratic PV bleeding in the first 7 days.
- If the patient vomits within 2 hours of ingestion, the recommendation is to take another pill of levonorgestrel (1.5 mg).

Further reading

FSRH clinical effectiveness unit guidance. *Emergency contraception*. 2012. Available at: www.fsrh.org/pdfs/CEUguidanceEmergencyContraception11.pdf

EMQs

Answers 1–3

1. H

Cerazette is a progestogen-only pill and its primary mode of action is inhibition of ovulation. If Cerazette is taken >12 hours late, i.e. 36 hours after the last pill, then it is considered as missed pill and an additional method of contraception (condoms or abstinence) is advised for the next 2 days or 48 hours after the missed pill is taken.

Further reading

FSRH clinical effectiveness unit guidance. *Progestogen-only pills.* 2009. Available at: www.fsrh.org/pdfs/CEUGuidanceProgestogenOnlyPill09.pdf

2. C

When switching from progestogen-only implants, injectables or desogestrel-only pill (Cerazette) to combined oral contraceptive pills, there is no need for additional contraception as both act by inhibiting ovulation. The pill can be started any time up to when the repeat injection is due or implant is due for removal or next day after the pill.

Further reading

FSRH clinical effectiveness unit guidance. *Combined hormonal contraception.* 2012. Available at: www.fsrh.org/pdfs/CEUGuidanceCombinedHormonalContraception .pdf

3. A

When there is detachment of a combined transdermal patch for more than 48 hours, additional contraception for 7 days is recommended. There is no need for emergency contraception unless the patch was detached in week 1 and unprotected sexual intercourse (UPSI) occurred in patch-free interval or week 1.

Further reading

FSRH clinical effectiveness unit guidance. *Combined hormonal contraception.* 2012. Available at: www.fsrh.org/pdfs/CEUGuidanceCombinedHormonalContraception .pdf

Answers 4–6

4. C

IUD is the most effective method of emergency contraception in comparison with hormonal preparations as antiretroviral drugs can increase or decrease the bioavailability of hormonal preparations due to the enzyme-inducing effects of some antiretroviral medication.

Further reading

FSRH medical eligibility criteria. *Summary sheets: common reversible methods.* 2009. Available at: www.fsrh.org/pdfs/ukmecsummarysheets2009.pdf

FSRH UK medical eligibility criteria for contraceptive use. 2009. Available at: www .fsrh.org/pdfs/UKMEC2009.pdf

5. C

Copper IUD is the suitable form of emergency contraception as this can be inserted up to 120 hours after the first UPSI or up to 5 days after the earliest expected date of ovulation. Ulipristal acetate should not be used more than once in a cycle and if it is more than 72 hours after the last episode of UPSI; hence, levonorgestrel emergency contraception is contraindicated.

Further reading

FSRH clinical effectiveness unit guidance. *Ulipristal Acetate (ellaOne°).* 2009. Available at: www.fsrh.org/pdfs/ellaOneNewProductReview1009.pdf

FSRH clinical effectiveness unit guidance. *Emergency contraception.* 2012. Available at: www.fsrh.org/pdfs/CEUguidanceEmergencyContraception11.pdf

6. J

As she is less than 4 weeks postpartum, an IUD is contraindicated. The most suitable option for her would be progestogen implant; as with Depo-Provera injections she needs to attend clinic every 3 months.

Further reading

FSRH medical eligibility criteria. *Summary sheets: common reversible methods.* 2009. Available at: http://www.fsrh.org/pdfs/ukmecsummarysheets2009.pdf

FSRH UK medical eligibility criteria for contraceptive use. 2009. Available at: www .fsrh.org/pdfs/UKMEC2009.pdf

Answers 7–9

7. E

COCP is the most suitable oral contraceptive option for this patient as it also alleviates her menstrual symptoms.

Further reading

FSRH clinical effectiveness unit guidance. *Combined hormonal contraception.* 2012. Available at: www.fsrh.org/pdfs/CEUGuidanceCombinedHormonalContraception .pdf

8. H

IUD is the recommended method of contraception in women with breast cancer as the breast cancer is a hormonally sensitive tumour and the prognosis may worsen with COCPs and progestogen-only contraceptives.

Further reading

FSRH medical eligibility criteria. *Summary sheets: common reversible methods.* 2009. Available at: http://www.fsrh.org/pdfs/ukmecsummarysheets2009.pdf

FSRH UK medical eligibility criteria for contraceptive use. 2009. Available at: www.fsrh.org/pdfs/UKMEC2009.pdf

9. D

The contraceptive options in this scenario would be transdermal patches or progestogen-only implant. Nexaplanon is a subdermal progestogen-only implant containing 68 mg of etonogestrel with the duration of action lasting 3 years.

Further reading

FSRH clinical effectiveness unit statement. *Nexaplanon.* 2010. Available at: www.fsrh.org/pdfs/CEUStatementNexplanon1110.pdf

Answers 10–12

10. H

Essure microinsert sterilization device is a coil-like device inserted under local anaesthesia into the bilateral fallopian tubes, where it is incorporated by tissue. After placement, women use alternative contraception for 3 months, after which hysterosalpingography is performed to assure correct placement. Postoperative discomfort is minimal.

11. I

POPs can be used for contraception when oestrogens or COCPs are contraindicated. They can be safely used during postpartum period and can be started at any time as they do not interfere with lactation or reduce breast milk. On the other hand COCPs should not be started before the third week postpartum because women are still at increased risk of thromboembolism prior to this time. Also COCPs can decrease breast milk. POPs are slightly less effective (other than Cerazette) than COCPs. They have failure rates of 0.5% compared with the 0.1% with combination oral contraceptives because COCPs mainly inhibit ovulation and POPs inhibit ovulation in only 50–60% of menstrual cycle and rely on alternative methods of action.

12. C

A copper IUD placed within 5 days of unprotected intercourse or ovulation can be used for emergency contraception and is almost 100% effective. An advantage of this method is that it provides continuing contraception after the initial event. Azithromycin 1 gm should be advised in such situations if the risk of infection is high.

Further reading

Guillebaud J. *Contraception: Your Questions Answered.* 6th ed. Edinburgh: Churchill Livingstone; 2012.

Collins S, Arulkumaran S, et al. *Oxford Handbook of Obstetrics & Gynaecology*. 3rd ed. Oxford: Oxford University Press; 2013.

Answers 13–15

13. L
Copper IUD mainly acts by blocking fertilization. It causes inflammation of the endometrial lining. Following this, the inflammatory cells in the endometrial lining appear to impede sperm transport and fertilization. One other mechanism described is phagocytosis of sperms; copper is known to be toxic to both sperm and the ova. Lastly, it can block implantation of the zygote, which is a back-up mechanism if the above mechanisms fail.

For emergency contraception, it can be used for up to 5 days after unprotected sexual intercourse and also up to 5 days after ovulation. This is more effective than levonorgestrel 1.5 mg. If the woman wants long-term contraception, various brands of copper IUDs can be used for the duration of 5–10 years without changing the device. One should warn the woman that her periods might become heavier than normal but this can be controlled with tranexamic acid in the first few cycles. Eventually this it may settle down.

14. I
POP can be used in women who are lactating and where COCP is contraindicated. It acts in several ways to maintain contraceptive efficacy. The following methods of action have been described which include (a) alteration in the cervical mucus or thickening of cervical mucus, which decreases sperm penetrability to ascend upwards in the uterine cavity; (b) inhibition of ovulation in 50–60% of menstrual cycles; and (c) reduction of the endometrial receptivity to the blastocyst, although this effect is weak.

15. G
Desogestrel (Cerazette) is a POP that contains 75 mcg desogestrel. Its benefits include inhibition of ovulation in 97–99% of cases, unlike POPs, which do this in only 50–60% of the menstrual cycles. Also, the window period is long (12 hours) when compared to POPs (3 hours). This is called the safety window and is more for Cerazette (desogestrel) than for conventional POPs.

Further reading

Guillebaud J. *Contraception: Your Questions Answered*. 6th ed. Edinburgh: Churchill Livingstone; 2012.

FSRH UK medical eligibility criteria for contraceptive use. 2009. Available at: www.fsrh.org/pdfs/UKMEC2009.pdf

MCQs

1A: False – Young women can be offered Mirena IUS even if they are nulliparous.
1B: False – If a woman understands the information given and is able to make an informed choice (Fraser competent) they should be provided with contraception. DMPA can be used in young women.
1C: False – Fraser competence can be assessed for women with learning disabilities as they may be able to make decisions of their own.
1D: False – Implants can be offered to young women who need long-term contraception and are not willing to take oral contraceptives.
1E: False – IUCD is not contraindicated in young women.

The long-term use of DMPA has been associated with loss of bone mineral density, although the exact effect is uncertain. Fraser competence is situation-specific and should be assessed carefully on an individual basis. Age and parity is no barrier to intrauterine methods (copper or Mirena IUS) of contraception, although possible failure of insertion and the need for screening for sexually transmitted infection should be considered when dealing with younger women.

Further reading

FSRH clinical effectiveness unit guidance. *Contraceptive choices for young people.* 2004. Available at: www.fsrh.org/pdfs/ceuGuidanceYoungPeople2010.pdf

Guillebaud J. *Contraception: Your Questions Answered.* 6th ed. Edinburgh: Churchill Livingstone; 2012.

2A: False
2B: True
2C: False
2D: False
2E: False

The World Health Organization (WHO) classifies contraindications into four categories:

- WHO 1: a condition for which there is no restriction for the use of contraceptive method
- WHO 2: a condition where the benefits of the method generally outweigh the theoretical or proven risks
- WHO 3: a condition where the theoretical or proven risks usually outweigh the benefits
- WHO 4: a condition that represents an unacceptable health risk (absolute contraindication)

The contraindications for COCP use include:

- Age >51
- Age >35 years old who smoke

- Cigarette smoking >40/day
- Severe or diabetic complications present (e.g. retinopathy, retinal damage)
- BP 160/100 on repeated readings
- Identified clotting abnormality of any kind
- Family history of a defined thrombophilia or an idiopathic thrombotic event in a parent
- Personal history of venous thromboembolism (VTE)
- Identified atherogenic lipid profile (family history of atherogenic lipid disorder or of arterial cerebrovascular event in a sibling or parent)
- Pregnancy
- Undiagnosed genital tract bleeding
- Migraine with aura
- Oestrogen-dependent tumours
- Active hepatobilliary disease or liver tumours

Further reading

Guillebaud J. *Contraception: Your Questions Answered.* 6th ed. Edinburgh: Churchill Livingstone; 2012.

Collins S, Arulkumaran S, et al. *Oxford Handbook of Obstetrics & Gynaecology.* 3rd ed. Oxford: Oxford University Press; 2013.

3A: True
3B: False
3C: False
3D: False
3E: True

Advantages and Disadvantages of COCP Use

Advantages	Disadvantages
• Reduces menstrual blood loss and pain • Regularizes the menstrual periods • Reduces the risk of benign ovarian tumours • Less incidence of PID • Possible less symptoms of premenstrual syndrome • Reduces the risk of endometrial cancer • Reduces the risk of ovarian cancer • Reduces the risk of colorectal cancer	• Increases the risk of venous thromboembolism (VTE) • Increases the risk of stroke (CVA) • Small increase in risk of breast cancer • A very small associated increase in risk of cervical cancer • Side effects: bloating, headache, nausea and fluid retention

Further reading

Guillebaud J. *Contraception: Your Questions Answered.* 6th ed. Edinburgh: Churchill Livingstone; 2012.

FSRH clinical effectiveness unit guidance. *Emergency contraception.* Available at: www.fsrh.org/pages/Clinical_Guidance_2.asp

Collins S, Arulkumaran S, et al. *Oxford Handbook of Obstetrics & Gynaecology*. 3rd ed. Oxford: Oxford University Press; 2013.

4A: False – Its use is contraindicated in women with breast cancer as these tumours can be positive for progesterone receptors.

4B: True

4C: False – Its use is not recommended in women with current DVT but can be used if patient has had a DVT in the past, depending on the rest their history.

4D: True

4E: True

Progesterone-only pill (POP)

[Levonorgestrel, Norethisterone, Etynodiol acetate inhibits ovulation only in 40–60% of women and has alternative actions] [Desogestrel (Cerazette) inhibits ovulation in 97–99% of women]

- Mode of action: thickening of cervical mucus, endometrial atrophy and inhibition of ovulation
- Indicated when the COCP contraindicated: during lactation, during puerperium, sickle cell disease, SLE and other autoimmune disease
- Side effects: menstrual disturbance (irregular breakthrough bleeding is common with POPs), headaches, nausea, mood swings, abdominal bloating, breast tenderness
- Interactions: it does not interact with broad spectrum antibiotics, rifampicin or liver enzyme-inducing drugs, which can increase its metabolism
- Window period
  - Is narrow (3 hours) and therefore should be taken daily at the same hour. If POPs are started on day 1 of menstrual period, no extra contraception is required.
  - If POPs are commenced after day 5 of menstrual period, extra contraception for 48 hours is necessary.
  - Missed POP rules: If >3 hours late or >27 hours since the last dose, then take last pill as soon as possible and take subsequent pill at usual time (extra contraception is required for 48 hours).
- If vomiting occurs within 2 hours after ingestion then take another pill and extra contraception is required for 48 hours.

Further reading

Guillebaud J. *Contraception: Your Questions Answered*. 6th ed. Edinburgh: Churchill Livingstone; 2012.

Collins S, Arulkumaran S, et al. *Oxford Handbook of Obstetrics & Gynaecology*. 3rd ed. Oxford: Oxford University Press; 2013.

5A: False

5B: False

5C: False

5D: True

5E: False

Failure Rates of Various Contraceptives Methods

Contraceptive Methods	Failure Rates
COCP	0.2–0.3% per 100 woman years
POP	0.3–4% per 100 woman years
Injectable depomedroxyprogesterone acetate (DMPA)	<1% per 100 woman years Given 12 weekly Side effects include menstrual disturbances, delayed return of menstrual periods, delayed conception (6–12 months), weight gain, bone loss
Etonorgestrol implant (Implanon)	<1% per 100 woman years Lasts 3 years
Vaginal ring (NuvaRing) Combination of oestrogen and progestin	Perfect user failure rate: 0.3% Typical user failure rate: 9% Duration effect: 4 weeks Inserted every 4 weeks It can be used for 3 weeks with a ring-free week or used continuously for 4 weeks, followed by change of vaginal ring, Releases 120 mcg of etonogestrel and 15 mcg of ethinyl oestradiol The disadvantage is it does not protect against STIs. Possible side effects include vaginal infection and irritation, spotting in between periods, nausea, vaginal discharge and mild headaches.
Transdermal patch (Evra) contains ethinyl oestradiol and norelgestromin	Perfect user failure rate: 0.3% Typical user failure rate: 9% Evra patch should be started ideally on day 1 of periods. If not started on day 1 of the periods then extra contraceptive precaution should be taken for next 7 days. Evra patch should be changed every 7 days for 3 weeks followed by a patch-free week. The break must not be longer than 7 days. Withdrawal bleed will occur during this break.
Levonorgestrel or Mirena IUS	0.18% per 100 woman years Lasts for 5 years Causes endometrial atrophy, thickened cervical mucus Menstrual blood loss decreases by 90% First-line management in women with menorrhagia Irregular PV bleeding common in beginning and therefore patients should be warned before insertion May be used in patients with history of breast cancer (oestrogen contraindicated) May be used in women who are breastfeeding May be used in patients with history of breast cancer (oestrogen contraindicated) but would depend on the receptor status of the tumour

Failure Rates of Various Contraceptives Methods

Contraceptive Methods	Failure Rates
Copper IUD	0.6–0.8% per 100 woman years Lasts 5–10 years Causes foreign body reaction and prevents implantation in endometrium Copper may inhibit spermatozoa motility Complications include heavy menstrual bleeding, risk of infection, perforation, dysmenorrhoea Contraindications include pregnancy, PID, active genital tract infection, uterine anomalies and copper allergy

Further reading

Guillebaud J. *Contraception: Your Questions Answered*. 6th ed. Edinburgh: Churchill Livingstone; 2012.

FSRH clinical guidance. Available at: www.fsrh.org/pages/clinical_guidance.asp

NHS Choices medicine guides. *Evra transdermal patches*. Available at: www. nhs.uk/medicine-guides/pages/MedicineOverview.aspx?condition = Contraception&medicine = Evra

Collins S, Arulkumaran S, et al. *Oxford Handbook of Obstetrics & Gynaecology*. 3rd ed. Oxford: Oxford University Press; 2013.

6A: True
6B: False – Levonorgestrel 1.5 mg (oral) should be ideally taken within 48–72 hours following unprotected intercourse to be more effective.
6C: True – It can be used more than one time during the menstrual cycle. However, it may not be effective. If the woman becomes pregnant during this period, its use will not harm or terminate the existing pregnancy.
6D: True
6E: False – Copper IUD is more effective for EC compared to levonorgestrel 1.5 mg (oral).
Either oral levonorgestrel 1.5 mg or the copper IUD can be used for EC. Levonorgestrel (Levonelle) is 95% effective in preventing unwanted pregnancies when taken within 24 hours. Its effectiveness falls to 60% when taken between 48 and 72 hours. It becomes less effective after this period. Copper IUD is almost 99% effective in preventing unwanted pregnancy and can be inserted up to 5 days after unprotected sex or after ovulation. However, it is important to prophylactically advise to take azithromycin 1 gm (oral) as these women are at risk of PID and will not have been screened.

Further reading

Guillebaud J. *Contraception: Your Questions Answered*. 6th ed. Edinburgh: Churchill Livingstone; 2012.

FSRH clinical effectiveness unit guidance. *Emergency contraception.* Available at: www.fsrh.org/pages/Clinical_Guidance_2.asp

7A: False – Current VTE is an absolute contraindication for use of the COCP. Therefore, the answer is UK category 4.

7B: True – Past history of VTE is also an absolute contraindication for use of the COCP. Therefore, the answer is UK category 4.

7C: False – Migraine with aura at any age is an absolute contraindication for use of COCP. Therefore, the answer is UK category 4.

7D: False – The answer is UK category 2 for migraine without aura at any age as benefits outweigh risks when initiating the use of the COCP. If a woman continues the pill, which was already in use, and develops a new medical condition, the category changes to UK category 3 (risks outweigh benefits).

7E: True

UKMEC

Category 1: no restriction of use of contraceptive method
Category 2: benefits generally outweigh theoretical or proven risks
Category 3: risks generally outweigh benefits
Category 4: unacceptable health risk with the use of a particular contraceptive method

Further reading

Guillebaud J. *Contraception: Your Questions Answered.* 6th ed. Edinburgh: Churchill Livingstone; 2012.

FSRH UK medical eligibility criteria for contraceptive use. 2009. Available at: www .fsrh.org/pdfs/UKMEC2009.pdf

8A: False – Oestrogen-only use is not recommended for contraception use during breastfeeding. However progestogen-only use while breastfeeding has not been shown to affect the breast milk volume.

8B: False – There is currently insufficient evidence to prove whether or not combined hormonal contraception (CHC) affects breast milk volume.

8C: False – Progestogen-only contraception has been shown to have no effect on infant growth.

8D: True – If women are in their first 6 months postpartum, amenorrhoeic and fully breastfeeding, the lactational amenorrhoea method (LAM) is over 98% effective in preventing pregnancy.

8E: True – In women using LAM, the risk of pregnancy is increased if the frequency of breastfeeding decreases (stopping night feeds, supplementary feeding, use of pacifiers), when menstruation returns or when >6 months postpartum.

Further reading

Guillebaud J. *Contraception: Your Questions Answered.* 6th ed. Edinburgh: Churchill Livingstone; 2012.

FSRH clinical effectiveness unit guidance. *Postnatal sexual and reproductive health.* 2009. Available at: www.fsrh.org/pdfs/CEUGuidancePostnatal09.pdf

9A: False – Women should be advised that contraception is not required before 21 days after childbirth.

9B: True

9C: False – If starting a hormonal method on or before day 21 there is no need for additional contraception. However, if starting a hormonal method after day 21, the clinician should make sure pregnancy is ruled out and should advise that she avoid intercourse or use additional contraception for the first 7 days of use [2 days for the progestogen-only pill (POP)], unless fully meeting LAM criteria, i.e. fully breastfeeding.

9D: False – Combined hormonal contraceptive should not be commenced before day 21 due to the increased risk of thrombosis.

9E: False – Women who are breastfeeding should avoid COCP in the first 6 weeks postpartum as there is insufficient evidence to prove the safety of COCP use while establishing breastfeeding. Women who are not breastfeeding may start COCP from day 21 postpartum. Between 6 weeks and 6 months the use of COCP is usually not recommended in fully breastfeeding women unless other methods are not acceptable or available. However, the benefits outweigh the risks in women who are partially breastfeeding.

Further reading

Guillebaud J. *Contraception: Your Questions Answered.* 6th ed. Edinburgh: Churchill Livingstone; 2012.

FSRH clinical effectiveness unit guidance. *Postnatal sexual and reproductive health.* 2009. Available at: www.fsrh.org/pdfs/CEUGuidancePostnatal09.pdf

10A: True

10B: False – Breastfeeding women should not start a progestogen-only injectable method before day 21 unless the risk of subsequent pregnancy is high. However, non-breastfeeding women can start this method at any time after childbirth.

10C: True – Women should be advised about the risk of this troublesome bleeding if injectable method is used during early puerperium.

10D: False – Copper IUD can be inserted within first 48 hours after childbirth in both breastfeeding and non-breastfeeding women. However, if this cannot be inserted within first 48 hours postpartum, insertion should be delayed until day 28 onwards. No additional contraception is required.

10E: True – An LNG IUS can be inserted from day 28 following childbirth in both breastfeeding and non-breastfeeding women. Women should avoid sex or use additional contraception for 7 days after insertion unless fully meeting lactation amenorrhoea criteria.

Contraception following childbirth

- Breastfeeding and non-breastfeeding women can choose to have a progestogen-only implant inserted before day 21 if this is convenient for them (outside the product licence for Implanon).
- The use of the diaphragm or cervical cap should be avoided at least 6 weeks postpartum before attending for assessment of size requirement.
- Women and men considering sterilization should be informed of the permanence of the procedure; about the risks, benefits and failure rates associated with sterilization; and about other methods of contraception including long-acting reversible contraceptive (LARC).
- Unprotected sexual intercourse or contraceptive failure before day 21 postpartum is not an indication for emergency contraception.
- Progestogen-only emergency contraception can be used from day 21 onwards and emergency copper IUD from day 28 onwards.

Further reading

Guillebaud J. *Contraception: Your Questions Answered*. 6th ed. Edinburgh: Churchill Livingstone; 2012.

FSRH clinical effectiveness unit guidance. *Postnatal sexual and reproductive health*. 2009. Available at: www.fsrh.org/pdfs/CEUGuidancePostnatal09.pdf

11A: True
11B: False – Women should be advised to use contraception while using infliximab or adalimumab and for at least 6 or 5 months, respectively, after treatment.
11C: False – Controversy still exists regarding the most appropriate mode of delivery following ileal pouch-anal anastomosis surgery.
11D: False
11E: True – Both men and women should receive appropriate counselling to optimize their IBD management prior to conception.

Further reading

FSRH clinical effectiveness unit guidance. *Sexual and reproductive health for individuals with inflammatory bowel disease*. 2009. Available at: www.fsrh.org/pdfs/CEUGuidanceIBD09.pdf

12A: True
12B: False – Women can be informed that a causal association between COCP use and onset or exacerbation of IBD is unsubstantiated.
12C: True
12D: False – Women with IBD using COCP should be advised to stop the pill at least 4 weeks before major elective surgery; alternative contraception should be advised.
12E: True

Further reading

FSRH clinical effectiveness unit guidance. *Sexual and reproductive health for individuals with inflammatory bowel disease.* 2009. Available at: www.fsrh.org /pdfs/CEUGuidanceIBD09.pdf

13A: True – All women with epilepsy should be advised before conceiving to use contraception until their seizures are controlled.

13B: False – If the woman is using hepatic enzyme-inducing drugs, double the dose of COCP should be used to increase the efficacy of the contraceptive pill.

13C: False – The dosage of POP can be increased to two pills per day and when the body weight is more than 70 kg it should be increased to three pills per day. This is unlicensed use of POP and therefore should be discussed with the patient.

13D: False – If she is taking hepatic enzyme-inducing drugs (primidone, phenytoin, carbamazepine, phenobarbitone) she should be warned about the need for higher doses of oestrogen to attain adequate contraception. When enzyme-inducing drugs are stopped, high-dose COCP and barrier contraception should be continued for at least 4 weeks since the enzyme induction continues for that length of time after stopping the drugs. The prescription of COCP falls into WHO category 3 (risks outweigh benefits) and UKMEC category 3. However, when a woman accepts the risks and declines other methods of contraception, one can use this method with extra caution. This is an unlicensed use of COCP and therefore should be discussed with the patient.

13E: True

UKMEC

Category 1: No restriction of use of contraceptive method
Category 2: Benefits generally outweigh theoretical or proven risks
Category 3: Risks generally outweigh benefits
Category 4: Unacceptable health risk with the use of a particular contraceptive method

Further reading

Guillebaud J. *Contraception: Your Questions Answered.* 6th ed. Edinburgh: Churchill Livingstone; 2012.

FSRH UK medical eligibility criteria for contraceptive use. 2009. Available at: www .fsrh.org/pdfs/UKMEC2009.pdf

14A: False – It is a permanent method of sterilization.
14B: False – The NHS does not offer reversal of sterilization operation.
14C: True
14D: True
14E: True

Sterilization Operation	Risks of Sterilization
It is an irreversible and permanent method of contraception.	The risk of failure rate per 100 woman years is 0.5% (1 in 200 women). Pregnancy can occur several years after the operation.
The regret rate is high when sterilization is performed in women who are less than 30 years old.	If there is a failure, the risk of ectopic pregnancy is high and she should immediately report to her GP for advice in the event of a missed period after the operation.
Current methods of contraception or abstinence should be continued until next normal period following the procedure.	There is a small chance of ongoing pregnancy even if a pregnancy test on the day of the operation is negative.
Sterilization is a minimal access operation. The fallopian tubes are visualized and clips are applied to both the tubes to block them.	The risks inherent in laparoscopy include bleeding, infection, injury to surrounding structures (1:1000 for bowel, bladder, ureter, and major vessels), postoperative shoulder tip pain, abdominal pain, embolism, failure to gain entry into the abdomen and unable to complete the procedure laparoscopically. The additional procedures include blood transfusion, repair of injured organs and laparotomy (open operation in the abdomen to deal with complications).

She should be fully aware of other methods of contraception including Mirena and vasectomy. Mirena IUS is as effective as sterilization and reversible.

Further reading

RCOG consent advice No. 3. *Laparoscopic tubal occlusion*. October 2004. Available at: www.rcog.org.uk/womens-health/clinical-guidance/laparoscopic-tubal-occlusion

Guillebaud J. *Contraception: Your Questions Answered*. 6th ed. Edinburgh: Churchill Livingstone; 2012.

RCOG other guidelines and reports. *Male and female sterilization*. 2004. Available at: www.rcog.org.uk/womens-health/clinical-guidance/male-and-female-sterilization

FSRH clinical guidance. Available at: www.fsrh.org/pages/clinical_guidance.asp

15A: False – If the girl is less then 16 years of age and has capacity (understands and digests information, makes an informed choice with all the information given to her without coercion) it is known as Fraser competence. She can be prescribed COCP.
15B: True – This method can be used if the girl prefers, although there are some concerns regarding bone loss with long-term use of Depo-Provera.
15C: True
15D: True
15E: False – She should be encouraged to inform her parents.

Further reading

FSRH clinical effectiveness unit guidance. *Contraceptive Choices for Young People.* 2010. Available at: www.fsrh.org/pdfs/ceuGuidanceYoungPeople2010.pdf

Guillebaud J. *Contraception: Your Questions Answered.* 6th ed. Edinburgh: Churchill Livingstone; 2012.

FSRH clinical guidance. Available at: www.fsrh.org/pages/clinical_guidance.asp

16A: False – COCP should not be used if a woman is continuing to breastfeed as this can affect both quantity and quality of the breast milk. In women who are willing to breastfeed, the progesterone-only pill is recommended as it does not affect lactation. It can be started as early as 3 weeks post delivery, in such women.

16B: False – In this case, she would definitely need emergency contraception in view of unprotected intercourse. Levonorgestrel 1.5 mg (Levonelle) can be taken up to 72 hours after unprotected intercourse, although its efficacy decreases with time. Women should be advised to take a further 1.5 mg if vomiting occurs within 2 hours.

16C: False – A copper IUD can be inserted up to 5 days after unprotected intercourse or ovulation. The Mirena IUS is not recommended or licensed for emergency contraception.

16D: False – Yasmin (ethinyl oestradiol/drospirenone) is a new monophasic COCP, which contains 30 µg of ethinyl oestradiol and 3 mg of drospirenone. Its anti-mineralocorticoid properties help to counteract the salt and fluid retaining properties of oestrogen and helps women who have symptoms of bloating, while its anti-androgenic property make it useful to prescribe in women with acne and polycystic ovarian syndrome. It can be used as an alternative to Dianette, which has been used in the latter condition. The anti-androgenic properties of Yasmin make it a useful pill to prescribe in women with acne.

16E: False – In this case, she should be offered a Mirena IUS before considering any other options. This should control the menorrhagia as well as provide contraception.

Further reading

Guillebaud J. *Contraception: Your Questions Answered.* 6th ed. Edinburgh: Churchill Livingstone; 2012.

FSRH clinical guidance. Available at: www.fsrh.org/pages/clinical_guidance.asp

17A: False – Depo-Provera injection is mainly used for contraception.

17B: False – It is administered 3 monthly (every 12 weeks) by intramuscular injection.

17C: False – It does not increase the risk of ovarian cancer but increases the risk of ovarian cyst formation. It also decreases the risk of endometrial cancer.

17D: True – Not usually recommended in the first 3 weeks following delivery as it can cause unscheduled excessive vaginal bleeding. However, it is safe for the infant as it is not secreted via breast milk.

17E: False – The return of fertility can be delayed by up to 3–18 months.

Further reading

Guillebaud J. *Contraception: Your Questions Answered*. 6th ed. Edinburgh: Churchill Livingstone; 2012.

FSRH clinical guidance. Available at: www.fsrh.org/pages/clinical_guidance.asp

18A: False – COCP can be used in women with migraine provided there is no associated aura.
18B: False – Heavy smokers above the age of 35 years are an absolute contraindication for use of COCP.
18C: True – COCP can be used up to the age of 50 years in the absence of other risk factors.
18D: False – If COCP is started on day one of the menstrual period additional contraception is not required.
18E: False – If COCP is started after day 5 of the menstrual cycle additional contraception should be used for 7 days.

Further reading

FSRH clinical effectiveness unit guidance. *First Prescription of Combined Oral Contraception*. 2007. Available at: www.fsrh.org/pdfs/FirstPrescCombOralContJan06.pdf

19A: False – The dose of levonorgestrel for emergency contraception is 1.5 mg (1 500 mcg).
19B: False – Levonorgestrel should be taken within 72 hours of unprotected sexual intercourse. However, the efficacy is increased (95% effective if taken within 24 hours when compared to 60% when taken after 48 hours) if taken within 24 hours of unprotected intercourse.
19C: False – Copper IUD is more effective (99% effective and can be used up to 5 days of unprotected intercourse) than levonorgestrel in preventing unwanted pregnancy.
19D: True – Only copper IUD is used for emergency contraception. Mirena IUS is not licensed for emergency contraception and is not as effective an emergency conceptive method.
19E: True – If the woman wishes to continue, then she should be allowed.

Further reading

Guillebaud J. *Contraception: Your Questions Answered*. 6th ed. Edinburgh: Churchill Livingstone; 2012.

FSRH clinical guidance. Available at: www.fsrh.org/pages/clinical_guidance.asp

20A: True
20B: True
20C: False
20D: True
20E: True

The 1967 Abortion Act

Abortion remains illegal in Northern Ireland, where the 1967 Abortion Act does not apply, but legal in the rest of Great Britain. Abortion is legal up to 24 weeks' gestation under the 1967 Abortion Act (amended by the Human Fertilisation and Embryology Act 1990). Two medical practitioners have to sign for the authorization of abortion. Under the Act, nurses are not permitted to sign the legal forms for abortions. Medical methods (oral mifepristone followed by misoprostol) can be used for termination of pregnancy up to 9 weeks (early medical abortion). In the UK, almost 90% of abortions are carried out by the 13th week of gestation. Surgical abortion up to 15–16 weeks should be carried out by trained professionals.

Further reading

RCOG: Evidence-based clinical guideline No. 7. *The care of women requesting induced abortion.* November 2011. Available at: www.rcog.org.uk/files/rcog-corp /Abortion%20guideline_web_1.pdf

RCOG briefings and Q&A: *The abortion time limit and why it should remain at 24 weeks – the O&G perspective.* Available at: www.rcog.org.uk/what-we-do /campaigning-and-opinions/briefings-and-qas-/human-fertilisation-and-embryology-bill/brie-0

Family Planning Association. *Abortion: your questions answered.* 2012. Available at: www. fpa.org.uk/unplanned-pregnancy-and-abortion/abortion-your-questions-answered

RCOG other guidelines and reports. *Termination of pregnancy for fetal abnormality in England, Scotland and Wales.* 2010. Available at: www.rcog.org.uk /termination-pregnancy-fetal-abnormality-england-scotland-and-wales